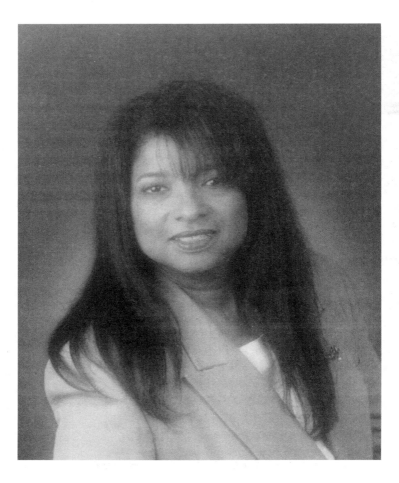

June 2000
Still growing 10 years later

Ultra Black Hair Growth II
Another
6" Longer 1 Year From Now

Ultra Black Hair Growth II
Another
6" Longer 1 Year From Now

Cathy Howse

UBH Publications, Inc. Denver

Published by **UBH PUBLICATIONS, INC.**
PO Box 22678, Denver, CO 80222
Copyright © 1990, 1994, 2000 by Cathy Howse

Ultra Black Hair Growth II
Another 6" Longer 1 Year From Now

Howse, Cathy
ULTRA BLACK HAIR GROWTH II
Another 6" longer 1 year from now

Library of Congress Catalog Card Number: 90-90326

ISBN 0-9628330-2-9

Revised and Updated

2000 Edition

This book is dedicated to my sons Greg and Brandon.

You can do anything you want; you just have to take action.

Acknowledgements

Hamilton-Sweeney Advertising - for their expert evaluation and advice

Copy Editors - Lila Burch, Ken Walker, Lesley Brandon, Terri Harmon and Josie Lund

Cover Photo - Leading Lady Photography – Shirlee Robinson – 10890 E. Dartmouth Ave Suite I Denver, CO 80014

June 2000 Photo- Shirlee Robinson

1989 Photo- Carlos Morales

Printing - Central Plains Book Manufacturing

Honorable Mention

Thank you Jehovah for allowing me to be used by you to get this message to our people.

Sincere appreciation goes out to the following people because without them it would have been a lot harder to accomplish than it was!

Diana Chaney, Craig Swank, Fred Scott, Henry Lardie

Table of Contents

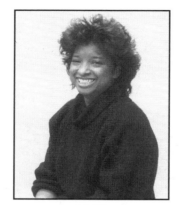

1987

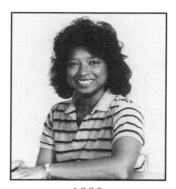

1989

Chapter One

Black Hair Care
A Common Sense Approach

Why are Whites, Hispanics, Indians, and Asians seemingly so fortunate to be able to grow long hair, whereas most Blacks have such a difficult time achieving the same? We want long hair too, and it is apparent by the surging hair weave business that promotes the slogan, "if you can't grow it, fake it." A hair weave, in most cases, constitutes a very drastic change, going from *no hair* to *flowing hair* overnight, but many women feel it is the only way to have long, beautiful hair.

We live in an instant world. The flick of a switch produces light. A frozen morsel popped in the microwave yields instant dinner. While wearing fake hair is an instant alternative, there is a more pragmatic approach to long hair. That approach involves applying common sense. You reason that all of your past attempts have failed to produce hair as "Sure Growth" products have claimed, so why should common sense be the exception?

Before *Ultra Black Hair Growth* was written, I remember wanting long hair so badly that I would try every thing to make my hair grow, but nothing seemed to work. Often, after trying a lot of the "guaranteed" hair growth formulas I ended up with a lot less hair. I tried "Sure Growth" products because, like all of us, we listen to the message they send in advertisements that claim to grow hair. Just like most ladies who have tried the same, I also got no results. The chapters ahead will explain why these formulas don't work and cannot produce hair growth.

The Myths

Most of our history of hair care information has been a series of myths, not facts. Perhaps you too have been a victim of incorrect information without even knowing it. The misconceptions that we follow hinder our hair lengthening options. We hear one thing, and then we read something else that is totally the opposite. We are confused because there is so much wrong information being circulated about our hair care. Shoulder length hair or longer for a Black woman, considering the dry condition that pervades, is no simple feat; it is a genuine accomplishment.

Behold one of the greatest hair myths:

"Trimming your ends will make your hair grow."

This statement is not correct because hair grows from the scalp, not the ends. Later in this book you will find out exactly who is perpetuating this myth.

> **When you trim off the ends, another piece of hair does not shoot out like a rosebush! Hair is not alive, but dead.**

Once the hair pushes through the skin, it is dead. If it were alive, it would be painful to cut it. Because it is dead, we need to stop saying things like "your hair can suffocate" or "your hair is thirsty." Get the idea about common sense now? By applying common sense, we help alleviate many myths associated with our hair care. The trick to growing Black hair is to apply common sense.

Another myth that haunts us is "washing the hair too much will dry out the natural oils." Water is moisture and can't possibly dry out hair. See the chapter on washing our hair and how this myth is disproved. (Chapter 4)

Ultra Black Hair Growth II dispels the myths by using a proven system for growing our hair longer. During my research to find the answers to growing our hair, I uncovered a wealth of information that we should know. Unfortunately, I found many untrue statements and myths that exist about our hair. Many product manufacturers are just as guilty about making claims about their products that are very inaccurate just to get you to buy a product! It is long past time to be ignorant where our hair is concerned; ignorance could cause you to lose your hair!

How Is Our Hair Different?

Ever heard the expression "hair is hair?" This expression happens to be very true. It means that all hair, no matter whose head it is on, has the exact same chemical composition or make up. It does not matter what race you are; the chemical composition of all hair is the same.

> **The elements that make up all hair are:**
> **carbon, hydrogen, oxygen, nitrogen and**
> **sulfur.**

Protein is also part of hair. If our hair is just like everybody else's hair, what makes it different? It's the characteristics that make each individual's hair different. Characteristics consist of color, texture, curl pattern and length. One characteristic that over 80% of the Black population has that distinguishes our hair from all others is the tight curl pattern. Scientific research proves that the curl pattern in our hair makes us have the driest hair of any race of people! It is really the excessive breakage caused by dry hair that causes our hair to look as if it is not growing even when it is.

> **The tighter the curl pattern, the drier hair will be.**

Extreme breakage is usually caused by the lack of moisture in our dry hair. Did you ever wear a curl perm or know someone who has worn one? What happened to their hair? Did it grow like never before? The reason for this astonishing growth was due to the constant replacement of moisture. Every day requires spraying hair with a curl activator solution when wearing a curl perm. The main ingredients in curl activators are glycerin, propylene, glycol, or sorbitol. These ingredients are humectants that absorb moisture from the air. Although products either can help or hinder our hair care problems, so can appliances.

Unknowingly, we do so many things to our hair that actually aggravates our dry hair condition. For instance; we blow-dry, iron curl, press our hair straight, relax it, color it, and perm it. None of these processes are individually damaging if they are done properly, or if the hair is properly maintained afterwards. But when you have a relaxer you want it as straight as possible, so you will most likely blow-dry as well. Blow dryers used to straighten the hair when it is not wet can mean immediate damage! Blow dryers used on a daily basis can also be very damaging for our hair. The excessive use of any appliance will result in lost moisture.

> **Our hair is unique in that no other race of people has hair as dry as ours.**

Because our hair is so different, our hair care products should not be geared to a generic market! This book discusses cleaning, conditioning, and moisturizing hair. It contains the information and treatments our hair needs!

Ultra Black Hair Growth II provides step-by-step guideline on how to maintain hair after chemicals, along with what nutritional needs are required to achieve longer lengths. All topics are applicable for our hair and only a few should be ignored. Pregnant women should already be taking vitamin supplements. For now it will suffice to read the chapter on vitamins, to understand why they are necessary. After your baby is born, and you are no longer on prenatal vitamins, then remember to follow the nutritional instruction.

Creating a moisture balance in the hair even when you don't wear a curl perm can offset a dry hair condition! By practicing a little common sense, you can help alleviate the majority of your own dry hair problems. Remember, you will always have some breakage. White people do too. The key to wearing your hair longer is to minimize the breakage!

Who Is This Book For?

Many Black women have at one time or another wished they could grow their hair but something always seems to happen that destroys that dream. Wearing wigs and extensions has never been an option for me because I have never liked fake hair. It is certainly okay to wear them if you feel comfortable. A number of women wear braids to grow their hair out. When you wear braids, every hair has a chance and is not subject to daily abuse and friction from our styling tools. But what happens when you want to stop wearing braids? How will you take care of your hair then? This book is for women who chose to wear braids then after they are removed it provides instruction and maintenance for hair upkeep.

Relaxers, curl perms, natural, color-treated, or any hairstyle may use this system. Relaxers are in my estimation, the driest chemically treated hair. Curl perms are only dry if they are not moisturized daily. This book is especially written for a dry hair condition, but not limited to only chemically processed hair. All people with chemically treated hair should follow this book. It doesn't matter if you are men or children. It may seem like a pain but keep in mind that this is a moisture balance system and if you use chemicals you are depleting your hair of moisture if it is not replaced.

I don't mention styling hair in this book. I believe you should be able to wear your hair any way you wish, within moderation, even if you use chemicals, and still be able to achieve longer lengths. Balding men and women ask me if this is for them. Balding can be blamed on side effects to medical prescriptions, illness and hormone imbalances, stress, menopause, thyroid disorders, diseases of the scalp, and age. If you have any one of these conditions this will not help you. Men, usually your problem with baldness has to do with testosterone. This book does not discuss baldness associated with hair loss caused by hormones.

This book does not address alopecia because there are many different types. It is hard to diagnose a balding problem if you don't know what someone is doing. Women will often experience similar balding problems as men. Some female baldness may be a form of temporary alopecia caused by wearing braids too tightly and the improper use of styling tools. Cosmetically induced balding caused by wrong or misapplied chemicals may also cause female baldness. These baldness problems are self-inflicted. This book will help problems of this nature, provided the hair cells inside the scalp are not dead.

Ultra Black Hair Growth II is for people with short hair that want to grow it longer. When this book was first published in 1989, Black hair growth was like a new science that very few had ventured successfully. Product manufactures knew what we wanted but failed to provide products and information to help us achieve the results we wanted. Products were marketed for our hair but research was based on what had worked with White hair products.

Not only is this book for Black individuals looking for answers about hair care and growth, this book was designed to teach all women and men how to keep the hair you have now and add length. It is intended as an instruction for Black teenage girls who have just started taking care of their hair. Young girls born of a mixed-relation, where their mother has no idea how to care for excessively curly hair, are also included. It is intended for every woman out there who has ever tried to grow her hair and could not. It is an instruction manual on hair care products and proper maintenance to keep what hair you have now and to add length!

Charting your progress will provide an accurate look at where you were, and what date you were there. If after one year your hair is still the same length as it was a year ago, then perhaps you have left out a step that is too important to be overlooked. Retry. This regimen is specifically designed to help you keep the hair you have now and assist hair growth.

Since this book can be read in one day, my suggestion is that you sit down and read it thoroughly before you do another thing to your hair! This is a reference book that you will need to refer to from time to time. Repetition will soon help you remember what you need to know about your hair. In fact, after you read this book once you should consider reading it again about once every month for the first year to be absolutely certain you are not leaving out any of the important steps required for growing your hair.

Keeping our hair on our heads should not be difficult. This book tells you how to keep your hair on your head. Learning to take care of your hair properly should be learned while you are young, no matter what style you choose to wear. Always having control will give you longer hair for a long time.

Why Should This Work?

Ultra Black Hair Growth II defines a moisture balance system for our hair to alleviate dry hair that breaks. The main objective of this book was to take the guesswork out of maintaining your hair when you have it chemically processed, which tends to dry the hair out more. Proper maintenance of any chemically processed hair will help you keep the hair you have now and add length, no matter how you style your hair. Proper care should be a requirement at all times. After you acquire proper knowledge of what to do, and what not to do, you can choose to wear your hair short or its maximum length!

This is a moisture balance system that you should use faithfully for one year. I believe you will be amazed with the results! This concept after 10 years is still like no other. Many books and web sites have sprung up in the last few years that claim to have the answers for growing your hair longer. Some are quite good while some are just another gimmick. Reading this book will help you identify the frauds.

To all you ladies and gentlemen who continue to write me giving your support for my work, I say thank you. I knew I had to be on the right track when so many of you responded favorably. Please continue to write me with your comments and success stories. I would love to hear from you!

UBH Publications Inc.
PO Box 22678
DENVER, CO 80222
ubhpublications1@covad.net

NOTE The subtitle, 6" longer 1 year from now is based on the fact that hair grows on the average of about 6" per year. The actual rate according to *Milady's Hair Structure and chemistry Simplified* (1993) is 0.01417 inches/day.[1] Although your growth rate may be average, the amount of hair you actually retain after 1 year depends on the natural life cycle of your hair and your hair's condition when you start this program. There is no fix for hair that has been severely damaged, except a pair of scissors!

---

[1] Douglas D. Schoon, Milady's Hair Structure and Chemistry Simplified (New York: Delmar Publishers Inc. 1993), p.52.

Chapter 2

The Professionals

Before **Ultra Black Hair Growth** was released in 1990, there were no truthful books about Black hair growth on the market. I expected a much different response than what I got from the hair care professionals. We finally had a proven Black hair growth system! Not a bunch of false claims as before, where Black hair growth problems were concerned. But, instead of being receptive about finally having the true answers to our hair growth problems, a great majority had opposing views! Over the past few years I found out why most of them were very negative. It is all about money. They want to be the authority. If you have to rely on them for all your hair care services guess whose pockets get fatter! It is definitely not yours. I am certainly not saying that the entire industry rejected my work, but there were many, many who did.

Doubting Thomas's

Believers reported astounding feedback about my hair care system from their hairdressers. Hairdressers all over were calling my hair a weave! Sorry folks, but I don't falsely advertise my hair products like the rest of the hair care industry! My system is proven. Based on fact, not fiction. Since I received so many comments like this when the first book came out, I thought it might be fun to share them with you. Some of the more humorous ones I've heard are listed below:

- "If you turn your customers on to that book, it'll cut into your money."

- "I can't use that stuff in my shop."

- One lady who had grown her hair out after 1 year of using my system (she showed me before and after pictures of her hair growth) told me a horrifying story.

Ida (not her real name) went to a hairdresser who specialized in curl perms. When she told the hairdresser about my book and wanted her hair treated as I had recommended, the hairdresser's comment was; "Yeah, you're not going to have to come in to the salon for treatments." (Insinuating that I promote women taking care of their own hair instead of going to the salon for treatments, which I do not.) She deliberately over processed, and did not neutralize Ida's hair, and she was devastated when she lost all the hair she had achieved after an entire year of using my system.

One of my distribution outlets requested that I remove the book from the store because it was not selling. The reason it was not selling is because the store manager was telling customers lies about the book. Someone later came back and told me she said, "I know that stuff doesn't work because I am a hairdresser." The clincher is the store manager who made the comment wore a ponytail wig!

Who's In Control?

Some hairdressers that did buy **Ultra Black Hair Growth** specifically told me that they would not share it with their clients for fear they would start doing their own hair. Please let me reassure, you insecure stylist. If people come to you for weekly treatments it is very unlikely that customers will change and start doing their own hair, unless the experiences have been so bad with you or another hairdresser that they realize that the only way to save their hair is to stop patronizing your business! In fact, I receive many letters stating, "My hairdresser was the reason I was losing my hair!"

I don't go to the salon for weekly treatments because I don't have that kind of money, nor do I have that kind of time, often hours, to sit around and wait for someone to do regular maintenance that I can do on my own. If you have $25.00 -- $30.00 per week to hire this service, go for it. If you enjoy the pampering and have time to spare, go for it. I operate on a budget and time constraints, so I have to be responsible for the way I look. I also have to know accurately what I can and cannot do to maintain my own hair, whether I go to the hairdresser or not!

The truth is, I need to be in control. Along with other women, I need to learn how to care for my own hair beyond salon treatments. I am not Oprah Winfrey so I don't have Andrea standing around in my dressing room waiting to do my hair. I have to do my own hair, as most women do and I need to know what to do and what not to do.

Gee folks, after hearing these comments I don't think I am the one you should be afraid of. You really should be afraid of the hair care industry because it seems the hair care industry wants to keep you in the dark! My intend with this book is to clarify how we as individuals should care for our hair based on what the industry offers and our specific hair needs. I want you to be able to make informed choices and not be persuaded by marketing hype.

Trimming Hair Ends – The Big Hair Growth Myth

Every other Saturday evening used to be hair-washing night for all the girls at my house. After our hair was washed, Mama would sit down and grease our scalps, brush the tangles out and section off little tiny areas for "plats" all over our head. We'd let it dry overnight before "pressing" it Sunday morning for church. Once a month Mama would also watch the full moon waste away with anticipation of the new moon to come, so she could "trim the ends of our hair to make it grow." Sound like the same ritual you're accustomed to?

No doubt the majority of Black women have had such scenarios drilled into their heads over and over again and probably never questioned it. As we grew older and wiser we began to ask, "How can that be true?" We reasoned that because an authority, usually Mama or someone in the hair care business passed it on, that it must be true. But can a dead hair end really communicate with the hair cell in the scalp?

Behold the truth about the trimming myth:

Trimming the hair does nothing more than even the hair ends and makes it look neater!

> **Since the entire hair shaft is dead, there is absolutely no way that taking the ends off the hair can send a signal to the live hair roots inside the scalp to produce longer hair!**

While sensibility disproves this statement, another woefully inaccurate myth about trimming is that untrimmed hair will split all the way up the hair shaft.

Just like the trimming to produce growth myth, there also is no evidence to my knowledge to substantiate that the absence of trimming hair ends will make it split all the way up the hair shaft. Split ends do not break evenly. Should your hair ends be split, common sense tells you it will break and tear off to the side before it would evenly split up the hair shaft. On the other hand, if your entire hair shaft is so badly damaged that there is a possibility that it can split from end to end, which is very unlikely, trimming the ends off will be of little significance anyway!

Trimming the hair is a maintenance step for appearance purposes only. Poor hair maintenance causes split ends. Often, once you stop doing so many damaging things to it like brushing, using excessive heat, and over-processing, split ends will be kept to a minimum.

Taking the ends off makes your hair have a neat appearance. But my experience has been that they usually take off too much. Have you ever gone to the hairdresser and asked for a trim and ended up with what looked like a cut? We've all had that experience. Many hair care professionals advise taking the ends off every 6-8 weeks. Some will even profess that taking the ends off, makes your hair grow faster! My suggestion is that you should not be so quick to get your ends cut off. You need your ends to obtain length and when you cut off the frizzy ones, you expose yet another end, only shorter.

One young lady that has beautiful long hair advertises that her hair products will help your hair grow. This young lady has beautiful long hair down to her waist. Her philosophy for growing hair is attributed to trimming. It amazes me how many people think this can be true. It simply does not make sense.

It is obvious this lady has done no research. She has long hair and is trying to capitalize on the fact that we want long hair. Just because she has long hair doesn't mean she knows anything about what causes or hinders hair growth! These gimmicks have been around since Madame CJ Walker. In *Madam C.J. Walker by A'Lelia Bundles* she mentions: *"On one of her frequent visits to Indianapolis, A'Lelia Robinson noticed 13 year-year old Mae Bryant... Because Mae had long, thick hair, Robinson thought she would make an excellent model for Walker products."*[2] After reading this book you will be able to spot the pretenders immediately. I wish I had a dollar for every time I saw celebrities promoting hair care products. Don't be fooled by celebrity endorsements. It's just another marketing ploy the industry uses to gain your confidence!

> **The truth is, cutting or trimming the ends has absolutely no effect on growth.**

---

[2] A'Lelia Perry Bundles, Madam CJ Walker (New York: Chelsea House Publishers, 1991), p. 53.

Trimming is necessary to correct uneven lengths remove split ends or broken hair. Remember, growth is controlled inside the scalp, not at the hair ends!

I never trim my ends. Occasionally, if it looks too uneven, I will have a trusted friend even it out. Trim it? No way! I know it is not necessary.

I deliberately do not trim my ends to prove that trimming has nothing to do with hair growth. It never has and never will!

Where Do Those Myths Come From?

It's hard to believe how often we are bombarded with myths. Even after ten years I still see where the majority of these myths come from. Unfortunately it happens to be the hair care industry. This book uncovers just a few of the ones I found during my research. The next section is not intended to offend, but to identify where we are getting our hair information and hopefully inspire change! It is essential for you to have factual information not myths to avoid wasting your money and to keep from damaging your hair.

Look Who's Talking

Be very skeptical about taking advice from fashion and hair care magazines. Unless it is about styling, the information is often wrong or ambiguous. Read on to discover some of the more humorous ones I found.

Barry Fletcher

In an article on hair Barry says:

> *"The winter season brings the use of hats and scarves which can sometimes suffocate the hair if worn too tight, too often, or if the fabric consists of wool.."*

Source: *Sophisticate's Black Hair,* May 1989 page 39.

Sorry Barry, but could you please explain to me how you can suffocate something that is already dead? Hair is not alive. This is very confusing information and very misleading.

LaVerne Powlis

LaVerne says in her book *Beauty From The Inside Out,*

> *"Split ends can stunt hair growth."*

No LaVerne, split ends have nothing to do with hair growth.

According to *The American Heritage College Dictionary*, the word *stunt* means to stop, control, or bring to a halt. Surely split ends cannot stop hair growing from the scalp, nor do split ends control the roots effect to produce hair growth. An interview published by a popular Black women's magazine stated that the information was gathered from hair stylists!

Source: *Beauty From The Inside Out A guide for Black Women* by LaVerne Powlis. Doubleday New York 1988 page 84.

An article entitled "Star Styling," in *Sophisticates Black Hair* November 1991 listed the following comments from top stylist about growing hair.

John Atchison

In the article John states,

> *"Regular trims and conditioning will help maintain the growth."*

Janet Zeitoun

In the same article Janet states under the subtitle, *Natural Growth, "Keep the ends trimmed."*

John and Janet I disagree with trims to "maintain growth." It is ridiculous to think that trimming hair controls hair growth.

Cynthia Taylor

The Ex-Beauty Advice Columnist for *Sophisticates Black Hair* in the Nov. 1991 issue states,

"Trimming or cutting the hair stimulates growth."

Sorry Cynthia, but trimming the hair ends has absolutely nothing to do with growth. Trimming off the dead ends can under no circumstances stimulate the hair cells inside the scalp.

Naomi Sims

In her book she states,

"It is not true, however, that our hair is any drier than that of other races."[3]

Sorry Naomi, but scientific research proves we have the driest hair of any race of people.

---

[3] Naomi Sims, <u>All About Health & Beauty for the Black Woman</u> (New York: Doubleday, 1976, 1986), p. 72.

Maybe we should do more research before taking these kinds of comments for granted. They are very misleading. These comments are false information directed at the consumer! No wonder we have so many problems, especially when we read this kind of information.

It kind of puts things into perspective when we view hairdressers as artists rather than scientists. They are in the profession of making your hair look good. Although hairdressers may be in a position of authority when you go to them for hair care, don't be so eager to accept these views and suggestions without question. Especially if what they are saying sounds suspect.

I have had hairdressers in my seminars actually try to logically convince me that trimming the hair ends makes hair grow. Their argument *appears* very convincing, but it is weak, and without scientific support!

Chapter 9 advises that you should no longer be brushing your hair. If you adhere to this advice, the amount of damaged caused to your ends by brushing will be diminished over time. Before you have the ends taken off, first consider sitting under the dryer with my special deep conditioner on your hair for 20-30 minutes. (Chapter 6) This should calm those unruly ends that are not split, but overly dry. Try wearing your hair in a style that allows you to pat the ends down, and in about six months to one year, have your ends trimmed.

The Authority

The hair care industry is actually perpetuating many of the myths we read and believe. We believe the claims must be accurate because they come from the authority! The product manufacturers who sell their products to hairstylist make erroneous claims about their products. Hairstylist, then regurgitate those false claims. Consumers should be skeptical about anything that sounds suspect. The industry is not concerned about providing you with accurate hair information. Their concern is the bottom line. The hair care industry must take responsibility for what is said just as any professional organization must. Otherwise, the authority is misleading us!

Paula Begoun had this to say about the hair care industry.

> *"The fundamental fact is that most hair-care companies don't tell you the truth about their products! Most hair-care companies make bogus or misleading claims about what their products can and can't do, and that can hurt your hair as well as your pocketbook. Because of this industry wide deceit, it is essential for every consumer to have more objective*

information so we don't have to waste money or damage our hair."[4]

Every profession has both good and bad people in it. The hair care industry is no exception. This statement is earmarked for the "bad ones." The best indicator of a good hairdresser is his or her own hair. If their hair looks suspicious, chances are you may be taking a chance with your own hair!

One shop owner told me the hair care business is on a need-to-know basis. "If you don't need to know it we won't tell you!" That is the biggest bunch of bologna I have ever heard. I see a hairdresser four to five times a year for a retouch, and nothing more. Logically, since my hair has to be cared for the other 360 days of the year, I want to know what to do to my own hair to keep it on my head and attractive all the time, not for just a few hours after leaving the salon!

> **Be very hesitant about following the advice of any person who is in the business of caring for hair if his or her own hair does not look cared for and healthy.**

---

[4] Paula Begoun, <u>Don't Go Shopping for Hair Care Products Without Me</u> (Washington: Beginning Press. 2000), p.8.

Since growing hair takes time to accomplish, it is really your responsibility to make it grow. Do not expect your hairdresser to perform miracles. You must perform the majority of the work to transform your short hair to long hair!

Identifying A Good Hairdresser

The first step in finding someone who offers a professional hair service and who will also respect your wishes is to ask around. When you have chosen a hairdresser, don't be afraid to tell them what **YOU** want and what you do not want. Have a picture of the style you like, if possible. Miscommunications have resulted in many unhappy people. If you know the terminology you can sometimes save yourself from bad surprises and hurt feelings. Don't go into the salon asking for a perm when you really want a relaxer. Know the difference between a trim and a cut. Ask questions before a hair service is complete. It may save you from disappointments later. You should not be charged for something you did not ask for. A good hairdresser will welcome your concerns, and advise you properly.

If you think the appliance being used is too hot, don't wait until your hair has been fried all over. Request that the iron be cooled down. It is your hair and you have every right to voice your opinion about the way someone is taking care of it. If you are reading this book your goal is most likely to keep your hair on your head!

Just like any business, the hair care industry thrives on repeat customers. When you find a good hairdresser, you generally express loyalty when you return for other services. Your hairdresser should be rewarded monetarily with appropriate tipping when your wishes are respected. After all, they are the "professionals" and you should give them a little motivation for doing what you ask. If they feel appreciated you can almost always be assured of getting what you ask for. You should also base your assessment on the quality of hair care advice and advice about hair products.

Buying Products

A sincere question asked by most salesclerks at a hair care center is, "Can I help you?" Never ask a salesclerk what she recommends for your hair. She is not paid to prescribe treatments for your hair. We are all guilty of going into these stores and asking impractical questions that cannot be answered by someone who has little or no knowledge of what type of hair you have. You should know your own hair. If you don't, how can you expect her to know? Hair is hair, but the characteristics of all hair are not the same. Most salesclerks are only programmed to direct you to a specific product brand. If they are paid on commission they might also guide you to products they can make more money on. They are not trained to address specific hair types and problems.

> **Know your own hair. Avoid taking chances.**

Product Reviews

Many of you have asked me how I feel about certain products. The two products that I have received the most recent inquires about are **Wanakee®** and **Copa®**. Since I have never tried either product I had to rely on other sources to help provide you with answers. Would I try them? I like my current products so I have no need to use theirs.

Wanakee —*Wanakee's Practical Guide to Hair* endorses the approach, *"Grow, grow, grow, trim – grow, grow, grow, trim- grow, grow, grow, trim. Notice, there's three times more growing going on here than trimming."*[5]

I continue to have great success with my method for growing my hair longer. My "common sense" approach will not allow

---

[5] Wanakee.com, <u>Practical Guide to Hair</u> (World Wide Web: 8/26/2000), p.1.

me to think otherwise. I firmly believe that trimming the hair ends has absolutely nothing to do with growth! It never has and never will. Most sisters can look at her hair and see her hair type is not the *typical* African-American Type 4. If you decide to read *Andre Talks Hair* by Andre Walker, you'll be able to identify her hair type as well as your own. Wanakee's hair does not appear to be Type 4.

Paula Begoun, author of *Don't Go Shopping for Hair Care Products Without Me,* had these comments to say about Wanakee products:

> *"The ingredients in the Wanakee products are just the same as those found in hundreds and hundreds of products made by other lines. There are good products to consider here, but Wanakee is not the final miracle for African-American hair-care needs."*[6]

Paula goes on to evaluate Wanakee products. She had this to say about her product **Advanced Conditioning Treatment.**

> *"Isn't all that advanced...It contains mostly water, thickener, slip agent, detangling agent/film former, preservatives, Vaseline, mineral oil, fragrance, and conditioning agents."*[7]

---

[6] Paula Begoun, Don't Go Shopping for Hair Care Products Without Me (Washington: Beginning Press. 2000), p.550.
[7] Ibid., p. 550.

Paula has this to say about her **Constant Care for Ends.**

> *"Is just thickeners and Vaseline. Plus, this is a lot of money for Vaseline and wax."*[8]

Paul goes on to say this about her **Oil for the Hair.**

> *"Doesn't actually contain any oil! It's just an extremely overpriced group of thickeners and slip agents. That can help when styling, and it is less greasy than other "oil"-type products, but this formula doesn't add up to more than 10 cents' worth of ingredients."*[9]

The opinions expressed by Paula are not the authors. I do not have a preference one way or the other on Wanakee's products. As I mentioned I have never used them. I continue to stand by my "common sense" approach to hair growth that obviously works for me.

Rio Hair Naturalizer System® —I know you all remember Rio. Rio was advertised in infomercials as being "all natural" and containing no chemicals. Sisters all over were devastated (not to mention pissed off) after they used this product and their hair fell out! Sisters used to ask me about Rio. Since it has been removed from the market, no one has asked me

---

[8] Ibid. , p. 551.
[9] Ibid. , p. 551.

about it lately. I inserted commentary about Rio because the FDA ruling on the product needs to be made known to those of us who prefer to wear chemicals.

Paula Begoun stated these comments in her book about Rio:

"In 1994 and early 1995, more than 3,000 people reported to the FDA that their scalp itched or burned and that their hair broke off or fell out—and, in some cases, turned green-after using the Rio Hair Naturalizer System and Rio Hair Naturalizer System with Color Enhancer."[10] Paula goes on to say, *"It was the largest number of complaints [the] FDA had ever received about a cosmetic product."*[11]

"Not only did Rio products contain almost exclusively a concoction of very unnatural ingredients, the pH of the relaxer was between 1 and 2, enough to eat through hair and scalp, which is exactly what it did. The rest is FDA history."[12]

"The company's labeling was false. The products' labeling listed an acid pH level of 3.4, but FDA and California State analyses of the product have found a pH range below 2. In addition, FDA that alleged the

---

[10] Ibid. , p. 174.
[11] Ibid. , p. 174.
[12] Ibid. , p. 174

labeling falsely described the products as "chemical free," even though the ingredient labels listed substances commonly recognized as chemicals."[13]

"Relying on the hair-care industry to give you the whole story about any product is rarely wise. Rio Hair is perhaps the extreme, but it is not the only case of blatant misinformation, lack of information, or misleading explanations about chemical content or product performance."[14]

Looks like I am not the only one saying the hair care industry is misleading, huh? Thank you Paula for telling the truth. Your work substantiates my research.

Copa Natural Curl Release System® —I have never used this product either and because I already have another relaxer product on my hair, I will under no circumstances change to try this product. I mention it here because sisters who use chemicals need to be informed about chemical options.

Paula Begoun in her book, *Don't Go Shopping for Hair Care Products Without Me,* had this to say about Copa.

"Depending on the type of hair you have (and how permeable it is) it can take from one to five applications ($19.95 per application) to achieve the

---

[13] Ibid. , p. 175.
[14] Ibid. , p. 175.

level of curl control you desire. In our testing, the average number of applications required was three."[15]

"Copa is very aware of the similarity between its product claims and that of Rio's because they take some effort to pinpoint the major differences between the two companies: "Copa uses sodium thiosulfate and Rio used acid and cupric chloride; [Rio had a] different active pH (Copa at 3.5, and Rio as low as 2; and Copa and Rio have different reactions in the hair (Rio [affected] the disulfide bonds directly and Copa has salt bonds). "[16]

Paula then goes on to evaluate Rio and Copa, and the claims made by Copa. In her book she then states:

"First, Rio did not use "acid." Rio used ammonium chloride, centrimonium bromide, and sodium thiosulfate, quite similar to Copa. Rio did have a very low pH, but the hair doesn't have something called salt bonds; the only molecular bonds that affect hair shape and disulfide bonds. If you don't break those and re-form them, you can't change the shape of hair, period. And there is nothing natural in the least about sodium thiosulfate. Rather, according to the

---

[15] Ibid. , p. 175.
[16] Ibid. , p. 175.

International Cosmetic Ingredient Dictionary and Handbook, sodium thiosulfate is the salt form of thioglycolic acid and is "used in hair waving and hair straightening products and depilatories." Paula ends by saying, *"So much for being special and different."*[17]

Again the opinions expressed by Paula are not the authors. I do have to applaud Paula for her research and insight. Although Paula is not a sister, her research is vital in helping us understand the hair care industry. The hair care industry is about money. It is unfortunate we as consumers are at their mercy. **Ultra Black Hair Growth II** together with Paula's book will make you an informed consumer!

Chapter Summary

1. There are good and bad people in every profession. Hairdressers are no exception.

2. The best indicator of a good hairdresser is usually how well his or her own hair is taken care of.

3. Trimming the hair ends has absolutely nothing to do with growth. It never has and never will.

---

[17] Ibid. , p. 176.

4. Know your own hair. Do not rely on just anyone to prescribe treatments for you.

5. There is an incredible amount of deception in the hair care industry. Don't be so quick to accept their ridiculous claims without question. Become an informed consumer!

Chapter 3

Black Hair Growth Facts

As Blacks, when it comes to wanting longer hair, we constantly question why our hair will not grow. What we really need to understand is that our hair does grow, but frequent abnormal breakage makes it appear as if it is not growing. If your head is bald or balding in an area of your scalp and hair does not return, then you can assume your hair is not growing. If it is not being cut, it is merely breaking as fast as it is growing!

This chapter will help you identify the most common causes of short hair on Blacks, and the cures I have found for these problems. As you begin to read the information outlined in this chapter, you may be surprised to find out that it is not only what we do to our hair that causes it to be short, but also what we do not do! **Before you can correct a problem with**

hair growth, you must first understand what the problem is!

Just The Facts

Fact 1   Hair grows on the average of about 1/2 inch per month. The actual rate is 5.17[18]. Some people may have hair that grows faster, others slower. For simplicity, lets say the average growth rate is 6" per year.

Fact 2   **Hair is not alive but dead!** What do you do to keep something dead? You preserve it! The keys to preserving hair will be explained in upcoming chapters. For now you need to know the essentials: keep your hair clean, have a proper moisture balance, have good circulation in the scalp area, proper internal nourishment, and an excellent maintenance program.

Fact 3   Scientists say the life span or natural life cycle of a single hair strand is 2-6 years, and your scalp can shed as many as 60-100 hairs per day.

---

[18] Douglas D. Schoon, Milady's Hair Structure and Chemistry Simplified (New York: Delmar Publishers Inc. 1993), p.52.

Breaking and shedding are two totally different matters. Shedding is part of your hair's natural life cycle. The old root is pushed out to make way for a new one. (Look for a little white bulb on the hair in your comb.) Breaking occurs when the hair falls off at a weak point in the hair shaft. If your hair does not break often, it can grow to be 12-36 inches long!

Fact 4 The curl pattern in your hair is what determines dryness. Scientists also say that over 80% of the Black population has dry hair because of the tight curl pattern. This partially explains the excessive breakage and shortness of Black hair when it is not maintained properly.

Fact 5 Cutting the hair has absolutely nothing to do with growth. Growth occurs inside the scalp at the roots. The hair you take off the ends is dead and logically has no effect on the roots!

Fact 6 The use of scarves, wool caps, and pillowcases does not break hair. Hair breaks because it is excessively dry or abused!

Fact 7 Hair is over 90% protein and there is no external product you can apply that will actually become part of your hair except another protein.

Comb your hair all over as if you are getting ready to style it, and look on the back of your shirt. Do you see lots of little broken hairs on your back? Are there lots of short pieces in the comb and on the sink? If so, then your ends are dried out and damaged. One of the most common causes of Black hair breakage! If you have this problem you must work fast to stop it. How to save breaking hair will be covered with more detail in the chapter on conditioning. (Chapter 6)

> **When the ends drop off excessively, length can not be accomplished.**

The longer your hair gets, the longer your ends have been on your head. The ends are what we need to keep attached to our hair in order to obtain length. Since the ends are the oldest hair, they suffer the most. This is the reason they break and drop off.

If your hair is 6" long and you wash your hair twice a week, your ends have been exposed to 104 washings. In addition to the drying factors of chemical processes, weather, and appliances, it is easy to see why we lose our dry hair in the absence of proper maintenance.

Common Causes of Breakage

The things we do to our hair can promote an overly dry condition and cause hair to break. Double processing is a major problem.

- Dyed hair that has been relaxed.

- Attempting to relax a curl style.

- Permanently curling relaxed hair.

- Trying to color permanently curled hair.

These are all combinations of double processed hair. Double processing occurs when one or more chemicals over another chemical are applied to the hair. Double processing is even more damaging than relaxers alone! Relaxers, hair dyes, and curl products are not designed to work together. When you combine hair treatments over each other, the hair is depleted of moisture and the result is breakage! Decide early if you want straight, permanently curled, or dyed hair. It is very difficult to have them all if you want longer hair!

Because there are so many myths about why our hair has its problems, I think you should understand that our choices are the real problem. To help identify the possible causes of your breakage, evaluate your hair care. Check the box to the left of each statement that applies to you regarding how you care for your hair.

☐ Do you use, or allow someone else to use, overheated appliances on your hair?

☐ Is a chemical relaxer repeatedly spread over all of your hair instead of exclusively to the new growth?

☐ Is the relaxer left on the hair after the comb out step, without immediately rinsing?

☐ Are you guilty of brushing your hair?

☐ Do you allow your hair to go for days without replacing moisture?

☐ Are you double processing your hair?

☐ Are you over-using heated appliances?

☐ Do you use instant conditioners every time you wash your hair?

☐   Do you allow your hair to go for weeks without washing it?

Looking over this list, how many did you check? Perhaps you have done some of these things for as long as you can remember. In fact, persons who have cared for your hair may have promoted some of these practices. Some of these statements may seem harmless to you, but be aware that any one or a combination of these further dry or abuse our already dry hair! If you are doing any of these things to your hair and you want to obtain length, your choices are the reason your hair is breaking! Any one item in the list can cause breakage and should be eliminated. You may be afraid to cease your practices, but the sooner you stop, the quicker your hair will recover. Your hair is breaking because it is too dry and brittle. To keep something that is already dry, you must think, "Preserve it!" To preserve our hair, we need products that work at alleviating dryness and a good maintenance program directed toward long-term preservation.

Products That Dry Out Our Hair

Before we can talk about products that dry our hair out, we must first understand the structure of a hair strand. (See illustration of a cross section of a hair.) A single hair strand has three distinct parts: cuticle, cortex and medulla. The cuticle is the top layer of hair that resembles shingles on a roof. It is in place to protect the cortex. The cuticle has no color. The second layer, the cortex, makes up about 90% of the total hair weight is what gives hair its elasticity, color, strength and flexibility.[19] Permanent products must penetrate the hair cortex. Finally, the medulla is the centermost portion of the hair that is usually only in thick, course hair shafts.

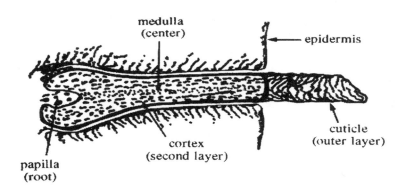

Cross Section Of A Hair

[19] Douglas D. Schoon, <u>Milady's Hair Structure and Chemistry Simplified</u> (New York: Delmar Publishers Inc. 1993), p.40.

Hair color

Hair color comes in three different forms: temporary, semi-permanent, and permanent. Temporary color does not chemically alter the hair but coats the hair surface. The two we need to concern ourselves with are permanent and semi-permanent. Semi-permanent color is similar to temporary color, but greater amounts enter the cortex as well as staining the cuticle. To be permanent, the hair color product has to lift the cuticle and penetrate the cortex of the hair shaft to change the color. Do you see why permanent color can be damaging? Both permanent and semi-permanent are chemical processes that can dry out our already dry hair more and should be used with extreme care. Using a semi-permanent color with relaxers or perms is okay. Frequent reapplication is necessary since it only stains the hair shaft it is gradually washed out in about 4-6 weeks.

Hair spray

The number one ingredient in hair spray is alcohol and alcohol is drying. Its purpose is to *dry* the hair into place. To *dry* our already dry hair is damaging. Hair spray should never be used on hair before using appliances. Hair spray was designed to hold your style after setting. Because of this product's ability to dry out the hair, I recommend you only use it when you intend to wash your hair the same day. If you decide not to wash it out after using hair spray to hold your set, be sure to moisturize your hair before going to bed to help counteract the drying effects. This product does not benefit our overly dry hair condition. Instead it encourages damage by making dry hair, brittle. My suggestion is totally avoid using hair spray if it will be a week or more before you wash your hair.

Relaxers and perms

Relaxers and permanent curls are chemical processes that can be both good and bad. They are good when they are cared for properly, and bad when they are misapplied and left un-maintained. Proper maintenance of hair that has been chemically processed is very important to help alleviate the drying effects caused by chemical processes.

Cathy's Dry Hair Care Program

Now that you are able to identify some of our common hair problems, I think it is time to share the hair care program that I have created to reverse our dry hair condition. *Ultra Black Hair Growth II* is a proven prescription for growing our short hair longer. At this writing, this system has been successfully tested and proven for over 10 years. This system works as a moisture balance that keeps our hair from drying out and provides an excellent maintenance program. Next are the requirements for my program, with exact details to follow in the succeeding chapters. The six requirements for Black hair growth are:

1. Frequent cleaning (Chapter 4)

2. Daily moisturizing (Chapter 5)

3. A conditioner that contains: protein to strengthen, oil to lubricate, and a scalp stimulant (Chapter 6)

4. Good blood circulation (Chapter 7)

5. Careful use of appliances (Chapter 8)

6. No hairbrushes (Chapter 9)

Step 1
Clean Hair

Chapter 4

Clean Hair

I remember as a child being trained to wash my hair every two weeks because I was taught that over exposure to water was damaging to my hair. Like many Black women the interval I was taught to wash my hair was every two weeks or once a month. When sisters wear braid styles, the time variation may be as infrequent as every three months! In the past 10 years I learned that frequent washing is not the problem, it's the myths and false statements we've been indoctrinated with that have proved the most harmful!

Many myths dictate our choices for how often we wash it. These myths were passed down from our mothers and our mother's mothers. The most popular one still alive today is, "Don't wash your hair too much because you'll dry out the natural oils." If that's not a false statement, what is? It really does not make much sense when you consider how frequent Caucasians wash their hair. The majority of them wash their hair at least once a day. If water actually dries hair out, they'd all be baldheaded! **Common sense tells us that water is moisture, and it is not how often you wash your hair that dries out the natural oil, it's what you wash your hair with!**

What Shampoo To Use

The basic job of a shampoo is to clean hair by removing dirt, excess oils, and scales. Shampoo formulations contain a number of ingredients that can help or hinder the physical appearance and chemical makeup of hair. Preservatives are ingredients naturalist shy away from but are needed in cosmetic products to inhibit the growth of mold and bacteria. They are also needed to give a hair care product shelf life. Without them, certain bacteria produce toxins that can cause blindness![20]

Conditioning shampoos —One characteristic that I do not recommend we choose in our shampoo is a conditioner. When conditioners are added to shampoo, the conditioner can

---

[20] Douglas D. Schoon, Milady's Hair Structure and Chemistry Simplified (New York: Delmar Publishers Inc. 1993), p.124.

interfere with the shampoo's ability to adequately clean the hair. While the shampoo is trying to clean the hair, the conditioner is leaving another substance to soften and smooth the hair. Essentially the dirt that you are attempting to wash out may be left on the hair when the shampoo conditions your hair.

Too much lather —Shampoo products that lather a lot are one of the biggest culprits in our fight to keep our normally dry hair from drying out more. Let's take a look at the lather produced by dish soap. Now raise your hand if you have ever used dish soap when you run out of shampoo. Don't be shy. We've all probably done it at some point in time. It pours like shampoo. It lathers like shampoo. If dish soap cleans dishes, then it should clean our hair too, right?

Any soap will clean just about anything, your hair included, but the problems we have when dish soap is used to wash our hair are: the product lathers too much, it has an alkaline pH balance, and is very drying. Soap is an alkaline product that can actually strip away the hair's protective layers that hold in moisture. Dish soap cleans dishes but if used on your hair it will strip the hair of all its natural oils and moisture. The same is true of shampoos that lather a lot. Avoid these types of products. A good shampoo must clean without stripping hair of moisture content.

Vitamins and minerals —Shampoos that contain vitamins, minerals, and all those other "essential" components are a waste of your money. These ingredients do nothing advantageous for your hair. The impact of these ingredients applied to the hair shaft has about as much affect as a mythical fountain of youth. The names on the product label suggest special qualities but do virtually nothing for hair.

> Protein is the only substance that attaches to the hair to become part of it!

The chapter on conditioners will discuss the use of protein in more depth. Vitamins need to be taken internally to influence hair growth. Nutrients are covered in detail in Chapter 7.

I have found that the best shampoo is one that contains an acid-pH balance, and formulated for dry hair. Don't worry so much if the product does not say pH balanced, on the bottle.

The most important requirements for your shampoo is that it must be specified for dry damaged hair, color treated hair or chemically treated hair.

If it contains all or any of these requirements on the label, the product should be the correct pH. Because maintenance products that we must use to add moisture to our hair have to be used regularly, buildups may occur on the scalp and hair. Buildups can look like dandruff and can be removed by using buildup removing shampoos or dandruff shampoos. These products are discussed later in this chapter. They work very well. Usually after the first treatment the once scaly scalp returns to normal. The downside for women who use semi-permanent color is washing your hair with any shampoo can prematurely remove some color. So frequent reapplication is necessary if you use harsh shampoo.

Is pH Important?

You better believe it is! It is very important to restore your hair to its proper pH after any hair process. The wrong pH in your shampoo can actually strip your hair of its natural oils and dry it out more. PH is a measure of how acidic or how alkaline a product is. The pH scale values range from 0 to 14 with the number 7 being neutral.

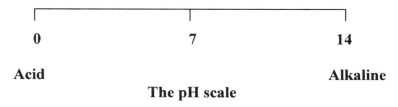

0	7	14
Acid		**Alkaline**

The pH scale

On the pH scale, numbers lower than seven indicate an acid solution. All hair falls between four and six on the scale and is naturally acidic. Numbers from 7 to 14 indicate alkalinity. A pH-balanced shampoo is slightly acidic, just like the natural pH balance of your hair.

Shampoos that lather a lot are too alkaline for our hair. High pH levels affect the cuticle that protects the cortex. Alkaline products actually raise the hair cuticle (outside layer of hair) and go inside the hair shaft. That's exactly what we don't want to happen to our hair when we shampoo. Some products have to be a high pH level to work, like chemical relaxers, and perm products, and permanent color. However, daily or weekly use of products with a high pH are very damaging to Black hair. Choosing an acid pH balanced shampoo will not deplete the hair of its natural oil, nor will it leave the hair without moisture.

To realize a visible difference, the pH would have to be either extremely alkaline or very acidic. Grocery store shampoo specified for dry damaged hair, color treated, or chemically treated hair is okay to use since many shampoos are now pH balanced. Having this insight should lessen your worry. But always keep pH in mind when choosing anything other than shampoo to clean your hair!

How Often To Shampoo

Frequent cleaning of Black hair is necessary because we must use hair products daily to help replace lost moisture. Daily moisturizing products (as discussed in Chapter 4) keep our hair from drying out. The moisturizing and oil products that we use attract dirt from the air, even though it is not visible.

Does your hair smell after a few days? Often it is because sweat and dirt have created bacteria on your hair. Together these two factors can cause hair to give off an offensive odor. This odor can usually be removed simply by shampooing. The use of a curling iron or other heated appliances can actually scorch hair and set the smell in it, especially if you use a daily moisturizer as recommended. Using an overheated appliance on hair that contains oil products is just like scorching grease on a burner, except you are doing it to your hair! Persistent scorched smells can be effectively removed with products that are called hair deodorants, which are sometimes used on hair after a perm to eliminate the chemical odors. These products work quite well if hair odors persist after repeated shampooing.

As far as frequency goes, forget the advice of our parents to wash our hair "every two weeks." Black hair needs to be washed about every three days. If you run into a busy schedule, washing can be pushed as far away as a week, but absolutely no longer than that. Every third day is recommended if you are just starting this program because you will need to deep condition your hair each time you shampoo to help get your hair in the best condition as soon as possible. If you wash more often than that, your frequency should depend on your life style. For instance, if you swim every day, I suggest washing your hair every day to remove chlorine.

After approximately three days, I have found that my scalp begins to get itchy. By the end of the week, if it has not been washed, generally my scalp will tend to become extremely itchy and scaly. When combing loosens the scales or when I scratch my itchy scalp, they cling to my hair unnoticed, which can be very embarrassing. My hair also becomes drier and more brittle the longer I go without washing it, although I have applied moisturizer as often as three times a day. Washing every three days to once a week is very necessary to grow longer, healthier hair. Never go beyond one week if at all possible no matter what style you wear your hair in.

How To Clean Your Hair

When you wash your hair don't pile it on top of your head. That's how hair becomes tangled after washing. Preferably, shampooing should be done in the shower so the hair stays straight during washing to do a thorough job. Massage the scalp very gently to help remove scalp flakes. After rinsing the shampoo out, apply the conditioning product described in Chapter 6, and cover your head with a plastic cap while you finish your shower. When the conditioner has been timed for deep penetration (as recommended), your hair must be rinsed well to avoid leaving traces of the conditioner.

How Much Shampoo To Use

Remember what the first sudsing of shampoo looked like when you washed your hair every other week? It usually had sort of a brownish hue to it. Right after that first rinse you probably didn't think it was really clean after seeing that so you put on a second application of shampoo and reworked it on the hair.

The more shampoo you apply to your hair each time you wash it will further deplete the hair of moisture and dry it out.

Usually the first shampoo will not lather a lot because of the oils on our hair, and that's okay. All we want to do is remove surface dirt anyway. One shampooing is sufficient, but two could be needed if you have been in an environment that is very dusty or dirty, or when you feel you've experienced a buildup of hair care products. If you wash your hair once or twice a week as the program advises in this book then one shampoo is sufficient each time you wash your hair.

Dandruff? Not So Fast

What you think is dandruff could be a buildup of maintenance products! Daily use of maintenance products can coat the hair, weight it down, and create scales on the scalp that resemble dandruff. Since we need to use maintenance products very frequently, one product you should become familiar with is clarifying shampoo.

Clarifying shampoos remove buildup on the hair caused by maintenance products. When you use a clarifying shampoo for scaly scalp, massage your fingertips gently across your scalp, especially in the area where the buildup is most prevalent. This will loosen the scales and allow them to wash away. Use a clarifying shampoo only as long as necessary. I suggest about every 6 weeks to get rid of product buildup. Switch back to your regular shampoo when the problem disappears.

People ask me why I don't manufacture a shampoo product. I have two reasons. My hair care system is not about how many products I can make and sell. It is about arming you with adequate hair care information to ensure that you make better decisions about your hair care. Second, there are already a lot of good shampoos on the market. Why should I reinvent the wheel? I do not use or recommend the same brand of shampoo be used for long periods of time, as the frequent changing of my shampoo seems to help control buildup.

Remember, water is an excellent source of moisture for our dry hair. Don't be afraid to use it, and use it often. Just be more selective about your shampoo, and use only products that don't dry your hair out when you wash it.

What Shampoo Products Do I Use?

Since my book was first published, I've received many calls and letters from people wanting to know what shampoo I use. Please do not think these are the only shampoo products I use. They are only listed here because people have asked me what I recommend. I have used Head & Shoulders occasionally when I have itchy scalp. I have used Neutrogena Clean and ION clarifying shampoo to remove buildups. I really do not have a favorite regular shampoo. I simply pick my shampoo product based on the specifications for dry damaged hair, color treated, or chemically hair. I have no problems with any product as long as the product label contains these

73

specifications. Since I use temporary color to cover gray, I look for gentle products that will not prematurely strip the color. Moisturizing, and humectants shampoos are good choices as they imply "non-drying." These descriptors are *not* a requirement.

Chapter Summary

1. Wash your hair every three days to one week.

2. Use a shampoo that is acid pH balanced and formulated for dry hair.

3. Be sure you rinse your hair well to remove any traces of shampoo.

Step 2
Moisturizing

Chapter 5

Do We Really Need Hair Grease?

Just about anyone you mention the name Madam CJ Walker to believes the first Black female millionaire made her millions by designing the pressing comb. In fact, it was not the pressing comb that made her wealthy, but the products she produced! One product Madam Walker made and sold was "medicated grease" called "Wonderful Hair Grower."[21]

Women who were using Madam Walker's techniques to press and curl their hair were putting this "medicated grease" on their scalp and hair, much like women do today, to keep from burning the hair when it was pressed. Three years later many

---

[21] A'Lelia Perry Bundles, <u>Madam CJ Walker</u> (New York: Chelsea House Publishers, 1991), p. 37.

of these women were reporting their hair to have grown as much as 16 inches.[22] Quite naturally, since most Black women had never experienced such phenomenal hair growth before, they began to assume that hair grease grew hair.

The hair grease had absolutely nothing to do with the growth, but a medicated ingredient was partially responsible for the increased length. Because most hair grease products contained a petroleum base, they helped prevent moisture loss in the hair, which in turn stopped their dry hair from breaking. I speculate that when people began to notice the success Madam Walker was experiencing with her hair grease product, numerous product companies and entrepreneurs also wanted a share of the wealth. That explains why we have such an influx of hair grease products on the market today!

With such an abundance of grease products for our hair, we often use them out of habit or because we were instructed to use them by people who cared for our hair. We wished and hoped for the claims of voluminous hair growth, advertised by the manufacturers of grease products, to someday come true. People please be advised. Hair grease does not grow hair! Remember the tingling sensation you felt on your scalp when you used sulfur and pine tar products? The smell was absolutely atrocious, but they were used because our hair

---

[22] Paul Giddings, When And Where I Enter The Impact Of Black Women On Race & Sex In America (New York: Bantam Books, 1984), p. 189.

seemed to grow better when we did. Do you recall the expression "stimulate your scalp to make your hair grow?" Well this is exactly what was happening! The stimulant in the products caused the hair cells underneath the scalp to produce more rapidly.

Hair: Dead or Alive?

The entire hair shaft is dead. The hair cells (roots) inside the scalp are the only living part of hair and every living thing must do two things: eat and get rid of waste. When the hair cells are stimulated, it causes them to do what they were designed to do all along. The stimulation was what enhanced the growth, not the hair grease product itself.

> **Hair grease does nothing more than coat the hair.**

Hair grease is not the answers to longer hair growth. A product that penetrates the hair shaft is needed for our dry hair condition and our chemically processed hairstyles.

Should We Oil Our Scalps?

We put too much emphasis on our scalps. The scalp is not our problem as far as hair growth is concerned. Oiling the scalp is not necessary because sebaceous glands exist on the scalp. The hairs oil glands secrete natural oil called sebum. Sebum, this slightly acid oil creates a coating that guards against lost moisture. Although this natural oil helps lubricate internally and externally the hair closest to the scalp, the moisture content is still lacking considerably at our hair ends. The ends, which are the oldest part of the hair, are the driest and in need of more moisture and lubrication than the scalp. A good hair conditioner will do for the ends of the hair the same thing sebum does for the scalp and the hair closest to the head. We do need oil to lubricate our dry hair. However, we do not need to grease or oil our scalps.

Oils that are absorbed into the hair shaft undoubtedly go where they are needed most, to the cortex (the innermost part of the hair shaft). Hair and scalp oiling may have been applicable in the past, but as the many ways to process hair continue to change, the requirements for our maintenance products must change as well.

The hair care industry was transformed with the advent of relaxers in the 50's and permanent curl styles in the 80's. We were transformed right along with them because we wanted to wear them. That's okay except the consequences of any chemical process to the hair exist whether it's a relaxer, permanent curl, or even just hair color. They all tend to exaggerate dry hair conditions. Although traditional hair grease products remain part of our culture for style and maintenance of Black hair, the moisturizing products that are formulated to improve a dry hair condition offer a more viable answer to our unique hair care needs.

The Need For Moisturizers

Most Black women and men inherit a biological trait that causes our hair to suffer from lack of moisture. The majority of our breakage is caused by this condition. The more moisture your hair contains the more pliable your hair will be. Another way of saying it is, the more moisture your hair contains the longer you can keep it on your head! Each time you relax, chemically curl, or dye your hair, the chemicals breakdown the hair structure and deplete what moisture it previously contained. Our hair needs moisturizers more than we need hair grease. Since water is the only substance that can moisturize, a good moisturizer needs to first contain water. Additional, it should contain oils to prevent moisture evaporation. Moisturizers are intended to replace the moisture over-processed dry hair lacks.

How Often Should You Moisturize?

All hair naturally contains moisture. Even dry hair has some moisture, just very little. Because of this condition we must use a moisturizer daily! I recommend twice a day the first three weeks after having a relaxer (or any chemical process), which is one of the times our hair tends to be the driest. At other times, a moisturizer needs to be applied once a day. If your hair feels drier than normal, you may choose to apply a moisturizer as often as three times a day.

> **Black hair should be moisturized every day — no exceptions!**

Crème moisturizers tend to feel greasy immediately after being applied, but after a short time our dry hair acts like a sponge and soaks up the needed moisture. The chapter on Clean Hair (Chapter 4) discusses the need for moisture to be applied frequently. When you use moisturizers your hair must be washed more often to avoid hair that separates because of excess oil and also to avoid odors.

Avoid saturating your hair with moisturizer at anytime. Moist hair is not greasy hair. **The absolute minimum you will need to moisturize is once a day!**

When To Moisturize

The only time it is necessary to immediately use a moisturizer is after you shampoo and condition your hair. Protein products that must be used to strengthen hair are also known to cause dry hair. A good moisturizer counteracts the drying effect. Use a moisturizer after washing and before you let your hair dry. Apply a moisturizer to your hair and ends. The amount of air-dry time will increase slightly but a moisturizer is necessary because it helps seal moisture into the hair.

As far as the time of day, you are free to use a moisturizer whenever you choose; night is no better than morning. In the morning, just before you have curled your hair for work or before you comb and style it, pour moisturizer in the palm of one hand; rub your hands together and lightly spread the product over all your hair. Application to each curl end with your fingertips is also a viable option. Make sure the moisturizer gets rubbed in to keep it from clumping on your hair. Using massive amounts of moisturizer is not necessary at any time, so use only enough to replenish the moisture content, without saturating. As time goes on, you will become more familiar with your hair and will be able to judge the correct amount of moisturizer your hair needs.

If you decide to apply the moisturizer just after you curl your hair, wait 10-15 minutes before combing so you do not destroy your curls. On days that you have not freshly curled your hair, a moisturizer still must be applied. A moisturizer's contents are damp and will flatten out your curls if too much is used and the hair is combed too soon after application. Proceed to style as you normally would after moisturizing.

Before going to bed, apply moisturizer to your hair the same way you would if you were to apply in the morning and leave it undisturbed for 10-15 minutes. I avoid applying then going right to bed. When I follow this method, the next day any curls I had the day before are usually still visible but maybe a little looser, unless it is time to wash my hair.

What Kind To Use

There are a lot of good moisturizing products on the market. At the time of my first two writings I believed the best moisturizers for relaxed and natural hairstyles were lotion-type professional products purchased at a salon or hair care center. I have since found that some sprays can also provide the hair with lost moisture without being too wet. The best moisturizer for braids and curl wearers is still a spray.

After 15 years of trying to find the right hair crème, frustration sent me back to the lab to develop my own. As of October 2003 my **Lotion Crème Moisturizer** is now available. Use Lotion Crème on natural, pressed and especially relaxed hair to help extend your chemical retouch.

Over the years I found out that not every woman who has relaxed hair wants to use crème moisturizers. I set out to find a spray that would work without weighing the hair down and that was not too wet. When I could not find one that I was happy with on the shelf, I decided again to make my own. I developed **Dew Moisturizer** to be used daily to replace lost moisture if you prefer a spray. Dew and Lotion crème are an excellent source of moisture for a dry hair type. A list of vendors who sell Dew Moisturizer and Lotion Crème may be obtained from the publisher. Visit our website at www.ubhpublications.com for instructions on how to order these products. To obtain a current price list or more information, you can also call 1-800-754-8751. Or send your requests to UBH Publications Inc, PO Box 22678, Denver, CO 80222.

Keep in mind that excess moisture increases the curl we just tried to eliminate. Spray moisturizers first ingredient should be water. I still suggest sisters with natural hair that has been straightened with the pressing comb use a crème moisturizer. I also recommend that products with protein not be used as a moisturizer because protein tends to dry the hair out more if applied at this stage.

If it looks like the first ingredient is grease or petroleum, put it back on the shelf! These products only coat hair. Black families have used heavy grease, hair oils and pomades for many years. We've been given the impression these products do something for our hair. Be advised that most hair grease does absolutely nothing but lubricate the hair, which is one of the necessary steps required for beautiful hair that is described in the chapter on conditioners. They should not be used as moisturizers!

Choosing a good moisturizer and using it frequently is required in this maintenance program. This step is second only to the conditioning step for increasing the length of your hair.

> **Successful hair growth must first stop breakage caused by dryness. A good moisturizer eliminates dry hair!**

Chapter Summary

1. Get rid of the hair grease. Grease does not grow hair.

2. Moisturize your hair everyday — no exceptions.

3. Moisturize immediately after you condition your hair.

4. Use a lotion-type moisturizer or a spray, depending on how you style your hair.

Step 3
Conditioning

Chapter 6

Conditioning

The signs of abused hair are lack of shine, split or frizzy ends, dryness, and excessive breakage. A good conditioner will work at correcting all of these problems. Conditioning is the external way to bring back healthy looking hair. It is also a preventive maintenance treatment and corrective medicine. Unfortunately, no conditioner will last forever once applied. Frequent reapplication is necessary!

How long has it been since you really conditioned your hair? I'm not talking about that stuff you throw on in the shower and rinse right out. I'm talking about the serious kind of conditioning you set under the hairdryer with for 15-20 minutes with a plastic cap covering your head for deep penetration. Furthermore, what condition is your hair in right now? You might feel it and say, "Not so bad." Do you even know what your hair feels like when it is in good condition? Chances are, you do not. You are so used to touching the same hair day in and day out that it probably feels "normal" to your touch. You say, "But I do condition my hair!" One very important rule to remember when you are assessing the condition of your hair is that just because the container says "CONDITIONER," it does not in fact mean the product is conditioning!

I will never forget the time I walked into the salon and told the salon owner, how I loved my hair since I had been having it professionally relaxed. He then replied, "If my hair felt like this I would be mad and probably not go back to the person who was responsible for this condition." Needless to say, what I thought was a good condition, really was nothing more than a slight improvement over what my hair felt like before. The improvement was next to marginal according to a different set of hands! Although, I thought my hair was in better condition, it really was not.

Our Need For Intensive Conditioners

As Blacks, the majority of us have the biological trait of dry hair and when chemicals are applied to it the condition worsens. The tight curl pattern in our hair is what determines how dry our hair is. In fact, over 80% of all Blacks suffer from dry hair and intensive conditioning is one thing that helps to correct this problem. Dry hair is also due to over-processing. Hair must be in top condition to grow beautifully. If your hair is like mine was when I first started my regimen, it is probably a long way from top condition. The one thing you have to look forward to is no unnecessary trial and error periods as I went through. One very important fact you need to know about extra dry hair is that it needs intensive conditioning!

Is your hair chemically processed? If so, hair care professionals characterize it as a dry, brittle condition after this process. The need for an intensive conditioner is mandatory if your hair has been chemically processed and you want to keep it on your head. Chemicals deplete the moisture in your hair. A good conditioner should pamper and protect the hair while working to strengthen hair by penetrating the hair shaft to help restore lost moisture.

Types Of Conditioners

There are two types of conditioners. They are instant conditioners and deep conditioners. The difference is that instant conditioners coat the hair, whereas, deep conditioners penetrate.

Instant Conditioners

Instant conditioners generally go on the hair and are rinsed out a short time later. The very small amount of this product that stays on your hair gives your hair a temporary shine and makes it easier for the comb to glide through. The majority of it washes down the drain in the final rinse. Instant conditioners, since they only coat the hair, give it the *appearance* of being in good condition. Most of these very light liquids contain wax to fill cuticle openings so light reflects off the hair causing a shine, making it easier to handle. When you choose to use instant conditioners, you have *temporarily* created the appearance of healthy hair. In most cases, you have done absolutely nothing to improve your hair's present condition!

Instant conditioners were used several times throughout my experiments when I ran out of my deep conditioner product. The results I received made me ban them from my regimen.

The results I experienced when I used them to condition my hair were:

- My hair showed frizzy ends within hours of washing

- My hair ends became quite dry and hard immediately

- More than average breakage resulted

Instant conditioners are not going to help you achieve that beautiful head of hair and they are NOT recommended for your deep conditioning!

Deep Conditioners

My research revealed that to get the maximum benefit from a conditioning product it needed to penetrate the hair shaft to:

- Strengthen the hair

- Provide lubrication

- And stimulate scalp circulation

Up until the writing of the first *Ultra Black Hair* book, to my knowledge there was no conditioner on the market that conformed to these requirements. The first of the three needed requirements, strengthening, may be addressed by the majority of deep conditioning products, but why not give your hair a hot oil treatment every time you condition also? Our excessively dry hair needs the lubrication that will be covered later in this chapter under oils. Lastly, since we should NOT use a hairbrush, which is covered in Chapter 9, we also need to find a way to stimulate scalp circulation that is less damaging to our hair. The best deep conditioner is one that does all three things.

Choosing A Conditioner

The trick in finding a good conditioner is, to find one that does everything our hair needs it to do. At the time of this writing, most product manufactures cater to a generic market —inclusive of both Black and White customers. Our hair needs are very different from our White counterparts. As mentioned earlier, even many products that are currently designed for Black hair still only address one or two of the real problems associated with Black hair, when actually it is a combination of problems that cause our hair breakage. Make it a point to remember that our hair needs a conditioner that strengthens, protects the hair by sealing in moisture, and stimulates. A good conditioner can be the prevention and the cure for a number of our external hair growth problems!

Now, how do you find a good conditioner? Here's a hint. If after sitting under the dryer for a deep condition and there is a lot of water in the bottom of the plastic cap, then certainly it is not on your hair and its contents are mostly water. Water will only condition your hair when it is present. When it evaporates, your hair is left unprotected! Since I was unable to find a conditioner product on the market with the qualifications I specified, I resorted to making my own.

Conditioner Requirements

The best conditioner for our hair should contain:

- Protein to strengthen

- Oils to lubricate

- And a Stimulant

The Strengthener

All hair is composed of over 90% protein and it needs protein to make it stronger. But incorporating extra protein in your diet will not directly help your hair. Instead, what you may see is a fatter body because your vital organs are more important than hair and nails and must be taken care of first. Hair and nails are not needed for us to live and even if they were both to fall off for some strange reason, you would not die. Right after reading an article that suggested that we should take protein supplements for hair growth, I began doing so, but soon had to stop when I became extremely fatigued. I found the cause to be the ingestion of too much protein. The brain uses up to 66% of all glucose circulating in the blood. According to Dr. Hatfield, when additional protein is introduced into the diet, it converts to glucose. As the body gears up for the extra fuel, very little is left for your brain.[23] I tired easily because as my body sped up to use the extra glucose, less food was left for my brain, causing it to starve!

A Need For Protein

Damaged hair and chemically treated hair is very porous and has the ability to absorb protein. When hair is damaged, protein is needed to help strengthen from the outside. Protein penetrates the hair shaft to provide elasticity and strength.

> **Protein is the only thing that attaches itself to the hair to become part of the hair!**

Protein is also very necessary to help control our breakage! Protein helps seal split hair thereby preventing the condition

---

[23] Frederick C. Hatfield, Ph.D., <u>Bodybuilding A Scientific Approach</u> (Illinois: Contemporary Books, Inc., 1984), p. 183.

from worsening. Protein conditioners are designed to penetrate to the cortex and replace protein the hair has lost. They also increase the strength and elasticity of hair.

When I applied a self-relaxer in June of 1989, protein was the only thing that actually worked at minimizing the breakage! Protein is needed to help save breaking hair and strengthen hair that is damaged.

The Lubrication

Sebum is the body's own natural oil made by sebaceous glands located next to the hair follicles. Each hair follicle has at least one gland and in some cases as many as six. The function of this self-made oil is to externally lubricate the hair and form an oil coating to prevent moisture evaporation. Oil is necessary because it helps to restore elasticity. Without it, our hair becomes stiff and brittle. A good moisturizer also contains oil to help seal the hair and prevent moisture loss. After years of being told to oil our scalp, the questions that remain to be answered are:

- If sebum's job is to lubricate our hair, do we still need to oil our scalp?

- Does oiling our scalp make our hair grow?

The answer to both these questions is NO! Press and curl styles made oiling the scalp popular because oil products were applied to the scalp and hair to keep the hair from burning during pressing and prevent reverting.

> **Oiling the scalp has absolutely nothing to do with hair growth.**
> **Grease does not grow hair!**

Oiling the scalp is not recommended because sebum, the hair's own natural oil, functions in that area of your hair. Oil in your conditioner actually goes where it is needed most, on the dry hair shaft to help lock in moisture and lubricate. If a conditioner containing oil it is applied to hair and heated with a hairdryer, the oil acts like a hot oil treatment, serving as a protectant by locking in needed moisture and lubricating dry hair. The excess oil is rinsed out when you rinse the conditioner from your hair, thereby leaving the hair moist and protected, not greasy.

The Stimulation

The scalp needs stimulation, and a hairbrush is NOT a good choice. Chapter 9 will discuss how brushing Black hair actually rips it off our head. Brushing should not be performed on our hair. The stimulation we need should come from our conditioner product. Hairbrushes were used in the past to "stimulate the circulation." I believe you should stimulate your scalp each time you condition your hair. Stimulation increases circulation in the scalp area. In order for hair cells to produce healthy growth, they must be fed and they must get rid of waste. Excess waste poisons the papilla and slows down the production of cells. Stimulating circulation in the scalp area will facilitate cell waste removal. Good blood circulation is promoted by taking nutritional supplements to feed hair cells as discussed in Chapter 7.

Ultra Black Hair Conditioner is now available ready made. It is the first conditioner that finally addresses African-American hair care needs. The product contains Aloe Vera protein for strengthening our hair, along with just the right amount of lubricating oils and an invigorating stimulant. A list of vendors who sell **Ultra Black Hair Conditioner** may be obtained from the publisher. Visit our website at www.ubhpublications.com for instructions on how to order the conditioner. To obtain a current price list or more information you can also call 1-800-754-8751.

Or send your requests to UBH Publications Inc, PO Box 22678, Denver, CO 80222.

How To Use The Conditioner

In the shower immediately after you wash your hair, squeeze off the excess water with your hands. Then put only enough conditioner to fully coat your hair, remembering also the hair at the nape of your neck. It too, must be conditioned, although it is under all your other hair and easy to forget. Braid wearers tell me they put my conditioner in a spray bottle and add water to dilute then spray it on their braids. After applying, put a plastic cap over your hair and finish your shower. Since this is a deep conditioning product, after your shower you will need to apply heat to your hair to allow the conditioner to penetrate. Heat causes the cuticle (outer layer of hair) to swell open, which allows the conditioner to go inside the hair shaft.

Although there are many methods for a deep conditioner, the hooded or dome-type hairdryers or the heat cap provides the best results. Stay in your robe because the best place to thoroughly rinse the conditioner from your hair is in the shower.

Timing The Conditioner

Heat is recommended for deep penetration because it speeds up the process. The least amount of time you can sit under the dryer and realize a deep conditioning benefit is 15 minutes. The conditioner and oils are not able to thoroughly penetrate the hair shaft adequately in less time. The standard time is between 15-20 minutes. If your hair is being pushed to the maximum time period on a retouch, (between 12 and 14 weeks), I suggest a minimum 20-minute conditioning time. (See Chapter 10)

You may reason that if a product says "leave on the hair for 20 minutes," that if you left it on for 40 minutes, your hair will get in condition in 1/2 the time it normally takes. That statement, unfortunately, is not true. The only thing that occurs is perhaps over conditioning. Over conditioning can make your hair limp and unable to style. Hair needs time and the proper environment to become stronger. Just like a broken leg, the bone requires time to repair. The cast creates the environment for that to take place. When you regularly deep condition your hair, the conditioner helps to create the perfect environment for beautiful hair growth! No matter what you have read or been told in the past, there are no "instant" or "miracle" cures for hair growth or repair!

Rinsing

When it is time to rinse out the conditioner, hop back into the shower to do a thorough job. Make sure you remove all traces of the conditioner because you do not want to leave any deep conditioning products on your hair for obvious reasons. Dried conditioners can cause breakage. Conditioner products can also buildup and even cause dandruff. Remember to also move your ears and lift your hair in the back.

Use a towel to blot the excess water from your hair and then apply a thin coating of moisturizer to it while still wet and allow it to air dry. I prefer to use my **Dew** moisturizer if I want a straighter style, and a crème moisturizer if I don't particularly care for a smooth texture. Moisturizer applied at this stage also helps seal the hair. You will find out later (in the chapter on appliances) why air-drying your hair is better for it. Do not allow your hair to dry without applying moisturizer, especially after you have just conditioned your hair with protein. Protein is very drying to hair when it is not moisturized, but as mentioned earlier it is also one of the requirements for having longer beautiful hair!

Chapter Summary

1. Use only deep conditioning products to improve the condition of your hair.

2. Deep condition at least once a week.

3. Use a conditioner that strengthens, lubricates, and stimulates.

4. Deep condition the hair for 15 to 20 minutes, using heat to cause deep penetration.

Step 4
Nutrition

Chapter 7

Good Blood Circulation

Everything we eat affects our body and our health. Even hair growth and quality is determined by what we eat. Because of this cause-and-effect relationship, it is important to know how vitamins and minerals help us to obtain beautiful hair. The condition of your blood circulating through your body has a direct effect on the health of your hair and nails. Since hair and nails are the least important of all our body parts and are not essential for life, they are the first to show the shortage when your body suffers a nutritional deficiency. When blood flow is poor, this can cause many problems including retarded hair growth and abnormal hair loss!

Take a look at your fingernails. Are they short? Do they contain white spots or black stripes? Do they break very easily? If so, this could be your body telling you that you need nutritional supplements. Not knowing that vitamins affected my nails when I first started taking them for my hair, I was surprised when a black strip disappeared from my fingernail that had been there for years! So did all the little white spots. Since the addition of vitamins to my diet, my nails also grow more rapidly.

Everything we do to our body affects it in some way. Smoking interferes with your circulation. The ever-popular crash diets starve the body, hair cells, and nails. Emotional stress and tense muscles restrict the flow of blood. Birth control pills are known to reduce zinc levels, and sugar depletes the body of vitamins and minerals. The more things you do that interfere with the adequate functioning of your system, the greater your need is for nutritional supplements.

Since I am not a doctor, I cannot prescribe nutritional supplements for you, although I will say they are very essential for beautiful hair growth.

> **The vital organs are cared for first. Hair and nails, which are not necessary for life, are the last to get any nutrients.**

One of the reasons hair grows so well on pregnant women is because of the addition of nutritional supplements to their diet, which are required for a healthy baby!

Good Nutrition

Every one of us probably eats on the run more often than not, and that cheeseburger and large french fry are certainly less wholesome than a meal representing the four basic food groups. Almost all of our foods are processed in some way. Even when we cook our food or prepare it for storage, nutrients are lost. We end up losing the vital dietary supplements that are required by our body for proper functioning and for beautiful hair. Natural foods, rather than synthetic foods, contain most of the necessary micronutrients and have more nutritional value, but how many of us eat all natural foods? I certainly don't. We need specific vitamins and minerals in our diet to facilitate certain functions. Without them, the cells of our body are not able to reproduce normally.

I take nutritional supplements for the following reasons:

- I do not always eat balanced meals

- I am still in my childbearing years and have a monthly menstrual period

- My body exhibits signs of anemia without them

- They facilitate healthy productive hair growth

Including nutritional supplements in your diet is certainly one way of assuring yourself that you are getting the necessary vitamins and minerals your body needs for growing longer, healthier hair. The Food and Nutrition Board of National Academy of Sciences establish the crucial vitamins and minerals everyone should include in their diet for a healthy body. A list of them can be found anywhere. The ones I have found to be important in obtaining longer, beautiful hair are iron and zinc.

Iron And Zinc

One of the biggest complaints I get when I tell people about iron needed in their diet for beautiful hair growth is that "iron is constipating." My answer to that statement is, take your tablets with some type of fruit juice and try eating more fruit to help flush your system. You might also choose chelated iron as it is supposed to be less constipating. One of the keys to hair growth is to make the cells reproduce at a normal rate.

Without iron in your diet, this process is hindered. Doctors have prescribed iron for years to women in childbearing years. Iron creates richer blood and is essential for the production of our red corpuscles because they carry oxygen to the cells. The cells can then live out their normal life expectancy of 120 days. Anemic blood does not carry enough oxygen. Without adequate oxygen, the cells will die prematurely. Remember that your hair gets the last pick of everything, including oxygen.

There is a high concentration of zinc in hair and a deficiency can cause hair loss. Zinc deficiency has been known for many years to cause hair damage in laboratory animals. Foods that normally contain zinc usually become deficient of this mineral when the food is processed. In some cases zinc does not exist at all due to nutrients lacking in the soil. My research revealed the necessity for both these minerals to be adequately supplied in your diet for beautiful hair growth.

Vitamin Supplements

If you now find yourself asking: "Can I get the proper dosage required for hair growth by just choosing to take a vitamin supplement with both iron and zinc in it?" My thoughts are yes. Any addition of a vitamin supplement that contains these minerals should be adequate. Iron and zinc require other vitamins to be present for adequate absorption. Nutrients not absorbed in the blood are simply wasted by the body. Instead of trying to decide which nutrients I lack, sometimes I will elect to take one complete vitamin supplement. The majority of the time, I purchase my iron in 18.0 mg and my zinc in 15 mg. These are the RDA (recommended daily allowance) set by the National Research Council, and consume one tablet each daily. Since these two supplements have an unusual after taste, I prefer to take them with fruit juice, to help conceal the flavor. Iron is also known to absorb best when Vitamin C is present in the body.

External Vitamin Treatments

Before you invest in hair care products that contain vitamins, you should be aware that: the external applications of vitamin products to your hair are of no value to it because all hair is dead. There are numerous product manufacturers who claim their ingredients restore nutrition to hair. Extensive tests performed on hair provide proof that hair growth does not come from putting a product on the hair or scalp. The papilla, located at the roots inside the head controls hair growth. So any vitamins that are applied to the hair shaft instead of the roots where growth is controlled are merely a waste of your time and money!

Precautions

As always, consult your physician before taking supplements of any kind. Iron can be harmful to persons with sickle-cell anemia or when administered in large dosages to small children.

Chapter Summary

1. Good blood circulation is necessary for beautiful hair.

2. Hair is dead and cannot be fed from the outside.

3. Iron and zinc are essential to hair growth.

4. Consultation with your physician or a nutritionist is recommended before taking any type of nutritional supplements.

Step 5
Careful Use
of Appliances

Chapter 8

Appliances

This chapter is intended to help you identify certain techniques you may currently be using regarding appliances. When I began searching for the answers to growing Black hair, I learned that the first deadly destroyer of our hair ends is the misapplication of chemicals. The second offender is heat abuse. The misuse of my appliances was also one of the reasons my hair was short!

All too often we become so used to seeing our face with a certain look when we use a blow dryer or some other heated appliance that we swear it would be disastrous to stop using them. I remember feeling the same way when I read about non-use of blow dryers after many years of use. Numerous articles would attest to the drying damages that could be caused by overuse. Although I often noticed excessively dry, frizzy ends when I used one, I felt I would have no idea how to style my hair without a blow dryer. Then one day it happened! I dropped my blow dryer, right in the middle of using it, and it quit working! Shocked beyond belief, I did make it through and to this day I use blow dryers very seldom. Determined not to run out and buy another, I decided to purchase a dome-type hairdryer instead and I began using it to deep condition my hair. This happened to be one of the greatest changes I could have made! My hair then had the opportunity to bounce back from its very dry condition because it now could retain more moisture!

Types Of Appliances

Hair appliances can take on many different shapes, sizes, and forms but one thing they all have in common is heat. **Heat is the worst enemy of our already dry hair!**

There are four appliances that deserve to be mentioned because their misuse can be causing the majority of your breakage problems and you might not even know it. They are:

- Blow Dryers
- Curling Irons

- Crimping Irons

- And Pressing Combs

Blow Dryers

This is not an instruction on how you should use blow dryers, but why they should not be used. Too much heat makes hair very brittle and easy to break, and results in lost elasticity. Some Black hair care professionals have suggested that we use our blow dryer on cool, but cool temperatures obviously will not straighten out our hair, which is usually one of the reasons why we chose to use blow dryers anyway. The only good thing that can be said about blow dryers is that they give the hair a more professional finish in less time. The bad news is that blow dryers range between 750-1600 watts and this excessive heat can damage hair even when used by a trained hairdresser!

After learning the damaging effects of blow-drying, and seeing how they strip the moisture and oil from our hair causing it to be dull, the only time we should use one is in emergency situations. For instance, if you are on vacation and you need to wash your hair the last thing in the world you would want to do is sit around waiting for your hair to air dry. Some women think that every time they wash their hair, it is appropriate to use a blow dryer, especially when they wait until the last minute to wash their hair before work, a date, or some other event. Evidence shows that air drying Black hair is the best drying method for it because the moisture we have just added to it by washing and deep conditioning will not be immediately depleted by intense heat.

Set aside a couple of evenings a week just for washing your hair so it has all evening if necessary to air dry. Avoid washing on nights when you know you may need to rush out to some evening function and air drying time will be impractical, if not impossible. When you air dry, the moisture your dry hair needs will last longer and so will the ends! If you need to dry your hair fast, try using your dome-type dryer on low or cool. The heat is spread out more evenly over the entire head, not concentrated on one area of the hair as in the case of traditional blow-drying.

Guidelines For Blow Drying

If you still feel compelled to use a blow dryer despite my warning, do not expect your breakage to be minimal. Follow these guidelines to minimize damage:

- Use the blow dryer on a low to medium setting.

- Do not dry your hair "bone dry." When you do, you not only remove the water, but also needed moisture. Without moisture your breakage is guaranteed to increase.

- Use a blow dryer only when your hair is wet, never between washings to straighten.

- Do not use a blow dryer on dirty hair. This appliance can actually cook or scorch dirt and odors into your hair.

- Maximum usage is once a week!

- Apply a moisturizer to your hair before using a blow dryer.

- If you notice lots of broken hairs on your shoulders when you comb out your hair after repeated use of a blow dryer, your hair is excessively dry and lacks the moisture to keep it from breaking. Discontinue use of this appliance immediately if you wish to save your ends and add length to your hair!

Curling Irons

Curling irons are another very popular hair appliance that also causes damage if used improperly. The two main problems that occur when you use a curling iron are that they are used too often and kept on the ends too long. Since I refuse to sleep on overnight curlers, the next option for me is to use a curling iron, and I consider it to be my most precious styling tool. It was after the removal of blow dryers from my weekly routine that I soon realized my hair was still too dry. After I learned what my hair should feel like when it was not dried out, I also realized that my favorite hair styling tool (the curling iron) was also causing damage. Due to the damage I suffered from using the curling iron, it became apparent that restrictions were needed with this appliance, too. The precautions I have found that work best when using my curling iron are very similar to the ones the hair care industry teaches, and I've outlined them below.

Curling Iron Precautions

- Always test your curling iron with a tissue or damp cloth before putting it on your hair. An untested iron can fry your hair in a puff of smoke before you realize what happened.

- Do not leave it plugged in longer than 10 to 15 minutes and expect to walk right in and use it. A curling iron will continue to heat up until it reaches its maximum temperature, or until something cools it down, either your hair or a damp cloth! If you happen to put the curling iron in your hair and it starts to sizzle or smoke excessively, remove it immediately and wrap a damp cloth around the barrel to cool it down. Be sure the cloth is thick enough to absorb the heat. If not, steam can escape causing scalding.

- Do not use a curling iron daily and do not use one on dirty hair. If you moisturize your hair daily, which is recommended in Chapter 5, your hair will need to be washed a minimum of every three days to one week maximum. This reduces curling iron usage to twice a week.

- Although blow-drying is not recommended, the curling iron, when used after blow-drying can be more damaging because of too much moisture lost between appliances without replenishment.

Minimal amounts of moisture can be re-added between appliances, but maximum retention of moisture is what your hair needs to get you through to the next washing and conditioner. The best precaution I can give you when using any heated appliance is to avoid abusive moisture loss from your hair at any time!

Straightening With The Curling Iron

When you wear a relaxer and you do not blow-dry your hair, it may still appear too wavy for you during certain times. I have found my curling iron has another function. Besides curling, it can also straighten hair! Your hair does not have to be totally straight in most cases, because you will have no body when you style, so a curling iron can be used to assist with straightening needs. The curling iron can straighten relaxed hair and new hair growth close to the scalp. Using this method causes less resistance, making the hair easier to manage, especially as you get closer to needing a retouch.

Straightening with the curling iron requires the same technique as curling, except you use smaller pieces of hair. Instead of winding the hair around the barrel of the curling iron, you pull it straight out. Once the iron has been tested, clamp it as close to the scalp as possible without burning yourself. Hold it at the roots for a few seconds when you have a lot of new growth, then move the iron slowly along the hair in a straight, outward movement. Apply this technique all over your head until finished. I acquire a smoother finish when I use **Dew** as my moisturizer with curling iron straightening.

Curling With The Curling Iron

We all have our own way of curling our hair with a curling iron. But, for those of you who may be open to suggestion, here is the best way I have found to use one. After the curling iron has heated up, take a small section of hair, wrap it around the barrel and time the section for about 10-20 seconds. If the curl does set after this period, proceed by finishing the rest of your hair using smaller sections. Larger sections are not recommended because we tend to hold the curling iron in longer for the heat to penetrate all the hair. At no time during use should the curling iron be left on the hair for more than 20 seconds. Holding the heated wand on your hair ends any longer than that is very drying and damaging to them. Not only can this appliance scorch the hair shaft, but it can burn your ends off as well.

Of course, we know that some curling irons do not heat as fast as others. If your curl flattens out or uncurls when you remove the curling iron, try repeating the heat up process time, leaving the iron to preheat approximately 5-10 minutes more before proceeding. Since less time may be required for some hairstyles, the maximum hold time you should keep the curling iron on your hair is still 20 seconds. Leaving it in place any longer will cause dry ends and can become the reason for more breakage!

Conditioning products or hair spray left on the hair can cause sticking when using a curling iron. If you have no choice and although the curling iron sticks to your hair, proceed with caution. The next time you wash your hair be sure you rinse your hair well. If sticking still persists, and you use a conditioner product that is left on your hair instead of being rinsed out, I suggest that you switch to the one I have defined in Chapter 6 of this book. Never use a curling iron or any other heated appliance when you have hair spray on your hair. Since hair spray contains alcohol and alcohol is drying, the use of one drying process over another is like adding fuel to the flame!

Crimping Irons

Crimping irons, sometimes called waving wands, are much like the curling iron except the concentration of the heat is not restricted to the ends. The wave wand can be less damaging because you only want a wave, and can merit great results in less time. The same precautions are advised. One alternative to consider is to braid your hair while it is damp or when it is dry, braid it and spray with a light misting of moisturizer to dampen, then leave it to air dry for a waved style that is less damaging.

Pressing Combs

Since this book was written from the viewpoint of relaxed hair, the pressing comb should never be used on chemically processed hair. They were not intended for this hair type. Often, a professional hairdresser will advise us to use the pressing comb when we want to go back from relaxed hair to our natural texture, or to switch chemical treatments. I still advise using the curling iron to straighten hair and new growth because the heat is not as intense as the pressing comb. I prefer to separate my hair with a wide-tooth comb or pick while it is being dried under the dome-type hair dryer because it helps to straighten the hair before using the curling iron to straighten.

For those of you reading this book that still have your natural textured, unprocessed hair, here is my suggestion. If you choose to have straight hair, you should consider using a relaxer. I too, was apprehensive about using relaxers until I learned how to care for my hair with one. After much research, experience, and years of using them, I am no longer intimidated. I have successfully learned how to care for relaxed hair.

As I stated earlier, to keep your ends you will need to moisturize daily. Press and curl styles revert too easily when moisture is present. The intense heat of a pressing comb will be required more frequently to keep the hair straight. You should not be afraid of using relaxers, unless you fail to take care of your hair after it has been chemically processed, or unless you have someone apply the relaxer incorrectly. My chapter on chemicals will instruct you on how to care for relaxed hair, explain what you can expect of your hair at various stages when you have one, and teach you how to keep relaxed hair on your head!

If you still choose not to get a relaxer and your desire is to have straight hair, then my advice to you is to only use a pressing comb with a thermostat control. The old fashioned kind that is heated on the burner, should be obsolete. That uncontrolled heat can easily destroy your ends and hair shaft very quickly. Remember, when the ends drop off your hair from damage, length cannot be accomplished!

Extra care is advised where extreme heat is concerned because the more intense the heat is from the appliance, the more moisture is depleted from your hair when you use it! Never put any heated appliance in your hair without first testing it. The extra few seconds it takes to test the heat of your appliance could mean the difference between straightening your hair and picking burned off hair strands from the pressing comb teeth!

Chapter Summary

1. Excess heat dries our already dry hair even more.

2. Blow dryer usage should be kept to a minimum.

3. Extreme caution is advised when using any heated appliance on our already dry hair.

Step 6

No Hair Brushes

Chapter 9

No Hairbrushes!

When I first started writing and researching hair growth in 1989, there was no prescription for successful Black hair growth. Every book I read mentioned, "Brush the hair." As children we remember being taught, "Brush your hair to stimulate the scalp and make the hair grow." We also probably remember watching old movies where the woman would sit at her dressing table, brushing her waist length hair the final few strokes of her 100 stroke routine before going to bed.

Hair care professionals for many years have also advised us to brush our hair. Naturally, after being repeatedly told all of our lives to brush our hair, we tend to do so without question. With everybody claiming this was true I reasoned, how could

I go wrong? In the middle of my research to write this book it occurred to me that this was wrong advice! Everyone seemingly has taken this advice for granted and very few have bothered to test the accuracy of this statement. Who would guess that a licensed hair care professional would be advising us to do something that would harm our hair?

Do we, as Blacks, need to brush our hair to make it grow? The answer is NO. History has given us three styles that prove brushing is NOT required for Black hair growth. They are:

- Afros

- Permanent Curls

- And Dreadlocks

All are styles that are not brushed, but have grown quite long on some people who have never had long hair, in their life. In order to grow beautifully long hair there is one rule that should be followed where brushing our hair is concerned.

That rule is: Avoid brushing our hair type at all!

Just for the record, brushing the hair can in fact stimulate the scalp, but it also damages and destroys the hair on our heads, especially if it has been chemically processed. Put aside all the myths about brushing our hair to make it grow. Brushing our hair does more harm than good!

> **Brushing our hair is one of the most damaging maintenance steps Blacks do their hair!**

If your hair is chemically processed either curl permed or relaxed, or natural and straightened with an appliance, and you choose to brush it, you can kiss your hair at the scalp and the ends good-bye. This technique causes too much stress on Black hair, and more so if you have chemically processed hair that is already weak and easy to damage.

> **Brushing the hair into a style is permissible. Repetitively brushing your hair from the scalp to the ends to produce stimulation will destroy it!**

Up until February 1989, I just could not understand why the crown of my head was balding in one spot. The culprit this time was my hairbrush! Exactly one year after I stopped brushing my hair, the bald spot had filled in with 6 inches of new hair! To those of you who may still choose to brush your hair despite my warnings, please consider the following arguments against brushing.

Arguments Against Brushing

The three functions of brushing were to: stimulate scalp circulation, to distribute the sebum oils from the scalp to the ends of the hair, and to loosen scalp scales and dirt. Brushing hair in the past was considered good for it. However, brushing our hair has no real value and is more damaging than beneficial.

- Stimulating circulation is necessary for hair growth, but hair does not need to be brushed to stimulate circulation. As we discussed in Chapter 6, products are available that can create this effect that are less traumatic for both the scalp and hair. The reason we need to stimulate circulation will be covered later.

- Since Black hair needs additional oil to lubricate it anyway as the chapter on conditioners tells us, any attempt to manually distribute sebum oil is not necessary.

- A good shampoo is formulated to loosen and remove dirt and scales, so brushing for this reason is also not a requirement. (See Chapter 4)

Brushing is very damaging to Black hair because of our curl pattern. The less damage you do to your hair when you care for it, the more you keep on your head. Remember dreadlocks cannot even be combed yet they grow quite well on lots of brothers and sisters.

Stimulating Circulation

The chapter on nutrition explained how the health of your hair is directly related to the condition of your blood circulating through your body. That is why vitamins are necessary for beautiful hair growth. Therefore, stimulating the scalp makes the blood circulate to feed the hair cells. Since hairbrushes should not be used on our hair, scalp stimulation must be achieved differently. Sufficient quantities of blood must reach the hair roots in the scalp to feed the hair cells because blood circulation is what brings food to the roots. If blood flow is inadequate or restricted in that area, growth can be retarded or not occur at all. Cells need oxygen to enable them to function. They also need nourishment and must get rid of waste. All living things accumulate waste and must eliminate it in order to function normally. Stimulating circulation feeds the cells and assists them in waste removal. The use of stimulating products in your conditioner as opposed to brushing is a better way of stimulating circulation. This method is covered extensively in the chapter on conditioners.

The Comb and Pick

To keep your hair on your head, you must always handle it with care. Pulling and tugging on it to remove tangles is very damaging to weak hair, especially hair that has been chemically processed. The less damage and stress we inflict upon our hair, the more we can keep on our heads! Using the wrong styling tool can also be damaging, even something so simple as using the wrong comb!

To avoid unnecessary pulling and tearing I have found we need a minimum of two combs and a pick to style and maintain Black hair. Especially if you wear it in a relaxed style because the texture changes periodically between retouches. One comb should be a standard size comb with large and small teeth. The other should be a wide-tooth comb. The standard size comb can be used on fine hair or only when your hair has been recently relaxed. If your hair "pops" and "pings" while being combed with the standard size comb, then immediately switch to the wide tooth to avoid severely damaging your hair further.

The pick or wide-tooth comb should be used to style your hair when the hair texture becomes tighter. I find when wearing a relaxer it is usually between 6-8 weeks. The pick or wide-tooth comb is less likely to get caught in tangles and rip out your hair. They should also be used on hair just after washing to separate the hair strands and lessen air-drying time.

My Experience With Brushing

Brushing my hair turned out to be one of the most severe mistakes I made during my entire testing and research period while writing this book. Because I was listening to what others were proclaiming, I practically brushed my hair off my head while trying to produce growth!

During the first year of my research I would brush my hair and scalp vigorously in an attempt to stimulate circulation. I brushed my hair from the time I got back from the hairdresser after a retouch, up until two weeks before the next retouch. Accumulations of hair would be in my brush, on my sink, and on my shoulders, but I thought nothing of it, since I was taking care of my hair internally with vitamins and externally with a good conditioning maintenance program. It was not apparent where the hair was breaking at first.

Numerous long hair strands in my brush made me reason it was part of my "natural life cycle" of hair loss. I never suspected this breakage to be abnormal. I noticed after about a year of this, the hair at the nape of my neck and around my temples was very sparse. Both were places I had brushed the hardest. My hair was being damaged so badly in some places that patches of hair were breaking off!

In February 1989, about a year after I started writing this book, I realized I was actually ripping my hair out at the roots and badly eroding the hair shaft! When my hair was retouched in March 1989, it was apparent that the breakage had occurred where I had brushed my hair the most. The left side of my head at the temple was no more than an inch long. There was a red streak on that side that I had hoped would get longer, so that area was brushed quite hard. The nape of my neck showed extreme breakage. Also, another area I brushed very vigorously in an attempt to make it grow longer was the back. My approach consisted of false ideas that I had adopted because I believed that brushing my hair was good for it.

Since the removal of brushing from my hair care routine, my hair now has a total fullness like never before. Actually it is fuller all over, even in places where I previously noticed thinning. The bald spot on the top of my head has grown in so well today, that no one would believe I was ever bald there. My hair ends also gradually showed less damage.

One very valuable lesson I learned about this procedure was although my hair was constantly growing, I was regularly breaking it off by brushing it!

Chapter Summary

1. Using styling tool that don't overstress the hair.

2. Avoid brushing Black hair at all!

Chapter 10

Chemicals

Veronica Chambers sums up how I felt about my hair, as a little girl. 'Good' hair is straight and preferably, long... 'Bad' hair is thick and course, a.k.a. 'nappy' and often short."[24] This is what I was taught and how I felt. I was born with what I thought was 'Bad' hair. Many women tell me they felt that way too. I now know I have 'Good' hair that I can make better. Chemicals are not for everyone. If you can grow your hair with chemicals and keep it on your head, think how much easier it would be to grow it using this system chemical free. If you don't use a chemical you can skip this chapter.

---

[24] Paula Begoun, <u>Don't Go Shopping for Hair Care Products Without Me</u> (Washington: Beginning Press. 2000), p.168.

With the advent of press and curl we were able to opt for temporarily relaxing our tight hair curls. The only problem with 'press and curl' hair is you can't wear your nicely coifed style long in humid conditions or you'll end up with a frizzy version of what you originally started out with. When relaxers were invented we could permanently change our curly hair to straight hair. We were also exposing our hair to the potential for excessive damage. The problem with relaxers is we often lose so much hair that they are hardly worth the effort to have straight, un-reverting hair. The costs may equal the total loss of the one thing that we women pride ourselves on most, our crowning glory: our hair.

How Do Chemicals Work?

The most common chemicals on the hair care market are relaxers, perms, and hair color. Here is what happens when you apply relaxers to your hair. The chemical applied to the hair causes the disulfide bonds (sulphur bonds) to temporarily break.[25] The hair is manipulated straight by smoothing the product with a comb or the hand. Curl perms also require the hair bonds to be temporarily broken then be restructured by wrapping the hair around perm rods to produce looser, more uniform curls. After the hair has taken on the new shape, a

---

[25] Thomas Hayden and James Williams, Milady's Black Cosmetology (New York: Delmar Publishers., 1990), p. 59.

neutralizer is applied to cause the bonds to reform into this new shape.[26]

A neutralizer is an oxidizer that stops the chemical action and brings the hair back to its proper pH. Four common neutralizers used by the industry to stop the chemical reaction are peroxides, bromates, perborates and persulfates.[27] Peroxide is the most common oxidizer used in neutralizers and is the reason we often get red hair over time when we use relaxers.

The timing, rinsing and neutralizing phases of any chemical are the more important requirements. Without these steps, chemicals and left over residues can cause unnecessary damage. Timing is important because permanent damage can result if the product is left on too long. Damaged hair where the chemical bonds are broken, is not repairable. Rinsing the hair will only bring the hair's pH down to about 8. A neutralizer must be applied to bring the hair back to the proper pH.

These steps are very important. Chemically treated hair can be worn successfully without excessive hair loss if done properly at application and maintained afterwards.

---

[26] Ibid p. 60.
[27] Douglas Schoon, Milady's Hair Structure and Chemistry Simplified (New York: Delmar Publishers Inc., 1993), p. 84.

Why Chemicals Promote Baldness

Relaxers have always been criticized because they tend to break hair off, in some cases all the way down to the scalp! Douglas Schoon says, "Chemically changed or destroyed proteins in the hair determine damage."[28]

> **Ignorance is the biggest problem we have when we chemically process our hair. Without proper knowledge, we cause many of our own hair problems!**

The chemical in the curl perm is Thio (thioglycolate). The chemical in a relaxer is most often sodium hydroxide. These two chemicals are not compatible together. Breakage occurs when the two chemicals meet on the hair. This is the reason why once you have a curl you cannot switch to a relaxer and vise versa. **Never mix these two chemicals together on the hair because extreme breakage is inevitable!**

There can be any number of reasons we lose our hair when we wear chemicals, but the two most common reasons are

---

[28] Ibid p. 14.

improper application of the product and lack of proper maintenance afterwards.

After the application of any chemical, make absolutely sure that a neutralizing shampoo is being used on your hair to bring it back to its proper pH. I know this sounds absurd but don't assume that your hair care professional is using a neutralizer. I found out that my hairdresser was not using one after my relaxer for an entire year. I was experiencing excessive end breakage but gave it little thought. It finally became apparent after another friend began experiencing extreme baldness on the top of her head and asked me what was wrong. After careful contemplation, I remembered seeing the bottle of shampoo on the counter that is used explicitly for regular maintenance, not for neutralizing chemical processes. We often assume that just because a professional has a license, that they are doing the right thing. Don't assume. Make absolutely sure!

The application of any chemical should never be done on double processed hair. Double processed means using permanent hair color on hair that has been chemically processed or, trying to put a relaxer over a chemical curl or vise versa. None of these products were designed to work together and can mean severe consequences for anyone that tries too.

What Is A Relaxer?

Relaxers virtually provide what I call a worry-free style. It means I don't worry about going out with a straight style and when moisture permeates the air, end up with an unplanned, frizzy version of what I originally started out with.

Relaxers are hair straighteners, not perms, and it pays to know the terminology. A relaxer straightens hair whereas a perm curls it. Relaxers are one of the most drying chemical processes we can do to our hair, but considered by those who understand them to be worth it! Most relaxer products in the past were made from sodium hydroxide, which is the technical term for lye. The industry, over the past few years, has been switching to non-lye based relaxers. No lye products are made from calcium hydroxide. It is still lye but just a milder form. Because they are applied close to the scalp, relaxers are considered one of the most dangerous chemical processes. As the relaxer straightens the hair, the chemical also weakens it. Even when relaxers are applied by a professional, damage can result. Care must be taken after the use of a relaxer product or any chemical process to minimize hair breakage.

Relaxing the hair requires the chemical bonds in the hair structure to be altered or changed. This process results in weakened or damaged hair. Breakage occurs when many of these chemical hair bonds are broken, especially in the case of a wrongly applied relaxer or one put on already damaged hair.

> **The less damage you do to your hair during any process, the easier it is to keep it healthy and on your head.**

It is my understanding that there is no way to repair or reform broken hair. Broken hair that does not fall off immediately will eventually fall off over time.

The pH Of Relaxers

The pH scale helps us to understand just how serious relaxers really are and how even the slightest misjudgment can cause extreme breakage! The normal pH of hair is between 4 and 6 on the scale. Most relaxers are alkaline products with pH between 11 and 13.5. Relaxers made with sodium hydroxide have a high pH of about $13.0 - 13.5$. Hair removers have a pH between 11 and 12. Lye has a pH of 14. These numbers are very important because they tell you just how close you are to totally removing your hair when you relax it!

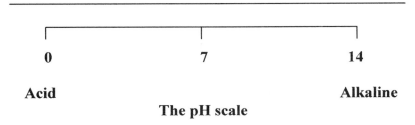

0   **7**   **14**

Acid   **Alkaline**

The pH scale

Repeated applications of chemicals to our hair decrease the hair strength and strip protein from the cortex.

Having hair relaxed professionally should not leave you concerned about the pH of your hair. The process used should include the necessary steps to bring hair back to its proper pH after any chemical application. It is necessary to be concerned when you do not have your hair relaxed properly!

The Relaxer Process

The purpose of a relaxer is to breakdown the curl pattern of the hair so it becomes permanently straight. Because of the chemicals used in this process, relaxers can damage your hair or actually dissolve it if they are wrongfully applied. The chemical solution is combed through the hair to soften and relax the curl. Once the relaxer has been applied, it is carefully timed to avoid over-processing, then it is rinsed out. A neutralizing shampoo is put on next to stop the chemical process, bond the hair into its new straight pattern, and return your hair as close as possible to its natural pH.

My advice is to be very careful if you attempt relaxing your hair on your own! Relaxers are very difficult to apply to your own head and the risk of losing your hair is greater when applied carelessly. Find a good hairdresser to do your relaxers. A good hairdresser does not overlap chemical processes. Overlapping occurs when the relaxer product is put on over hair that has been previously processed with a chemical.

Since all relaxer products are not the same, find out what product was used and try to stick with it! If you are a regular customer with the same hairdresser, they should remember what they used on you hair. If for some reason you decide to change hairdressers, be sure and request the same relaxer that was used on your hair previously.

The person applying a relaxer has to work fast because the relaxer product needs to be completely applied in approximately 10 minutes. After this time period, the straightening process begins. The next 15 minutes should be spent combing the product through the hair and then it should be thoroughly rinsed out immediately after comb out. Relaxers have timing guides that should be followed. Leaving it on longer than the specified time limit is very drying and can cause unnecessary damage to the hair.

Extensive rinsing is required to remove all traces of a relaxer product. The rinsing phase is one step where most self-relaxers suffer. The main idea behind extensive rinsing is to remove as much of the chemical as possible before shampooing. The neutralizing shampoo is applied afterwards to stabilize the process and reform the hair.

After stabilizing, caring for your newly relaxed style must begin immediately. A reconstructor should be applied now to begin the rebuilding process. The best conditioner to use after that step is the one I have developed in Chapter 6.

After conditioning is complete, I generally choose to towel blot my hair to remove excess water, and let my hair air-dry. The relaxer I've used for the past 10 years although it is still made by the same manufacturer recently developed a different form of the relaxer. The product instructions also changed. The neutralizer is now applied after 5 minutes of conditioning. There possibly are hidden benefits in conditioning before neutralizing but I'm too skeptical to find out. I strongly believe in neutralizing immediately after rinsing any chemical. Regardless of what the manufacturer says I prefer to bring my hair back to the proper pH immediately before conditioning.

The Retouch

A retouch is the straightening of the hair closest to the scalp that has grown since your last relaxer. As new growth is visible within 5-6 weeks in some people and 8-10 weeks in others, consider having a retouch of only the new growth. During a retouch, the relaxer product should not be applied from the scalp to ends of the hair. The only exception is once or twice a year to straighten previously relaxed hair that has regained too much curl. This exception can be very damaging and discretion is advised. Even so, the product still should only be combed through the new growth. I have found that each time the relaxer product is rinsed out of my hair, even if the chemical was applied only to the new growth, the previously relaxed hair responds to the chemical and softens again.

Repeatedly applying a relaxer over all your hair again is over-processing. Hair that has been processed by any chemical is already weak, considered dry, and prone to breakage. Remember, the less damage you do to your hair during any hair service, the more you will be able to keep on your head to add length!

How often you have a chemical retouch has been specified by the industry as 5-6 weeks or in some cases 6-8 weeks with good reason. I base the time between my relaxers on how much new growth I have and whether or not my hair is breaking unnecessarily. You really don't want to overuse any chemical that is applied that close to the scalp too often because these chemicals can penetrate the scalp. The scalp and skin serve as a protective barrier that somewhat repels chemicals, but it is not a fortress. This is evidenced by nicotine patches applied to the skin as a deterrent for smokers. Nicotine enters the body through the skin. Therefore frequent application of chemicals can also penetrate. Keep in mind the less frequency you use when you apply chemicals to your hair, the better off your hair will be.

The average time period for a retouch varies with the individual. I have had people tell me they only get a relaxer twice a year. Remember some people have hair that grows faster than others. My experience has been that retouches can be extended without severe breakage if you have a good maintenance program. Measuring growth is somewhat difficult to do because of the curl pattern in our hair. I have found that measuring after the retouch is truer, and then base your retouches on the amount of time it took to obtain a certain amount of growth. It takes me 12-14 weeks to obtain 1-½ inches of new growth, which equates to about 1 inch of hair every two months or approximately 6" per year.

If you condition with my conditioner product described in Chapter 5, for 30 minutes under the dryer, allow it to air dry with a moisturizer on it, then straighten with the curling iron, you may also be able to avoid having a retouch for as long as 3 months. This is not a requirement, just a suggestion.

Before The Retouch

The morning before my retouch I always make sure I moisturize my hair to help protect it from over drying. I also will try to set my hair appointments for a retouch on Friday evening after work and try to avoid using any heated appliances until Monday morning when I have to get ready for my job. During the weekend, after my hair has been chemically processed, I moisturize constantly to help replace lost moisture. Since your schedule may be different from mine this may not work for you. Just remember that relaxers and appliances dry our already dry hair. The best immediate option for your hair is to avoid doing too many unnecessary processes to it until it has at least a couple of days to regain lost moisture!

Caring For Relaxed Hair

The application of any chemical process strips the hair of moisture content and impairs the natural structure of the hair shaft. If you want to keep your hair on your head after any chemical has been applied, the priority is to keep it soft and to replace lost moisture! Even after rinsing a relaxer product from your hair, the pH of your hair is still about 10. Relaxers are less damaging if you know how to care for your hair after your treatment. Before you attempt to put that new straight hair into a style, I recommend that for the first two weeks after you have your relaxer or retouch, you sit under the dryer with a good conditioner for at least 20-30 minutes each time you wash your hair. And everyday, without exception, you must moisturize!

> **One of the reasons we lose our hair after a relaxer is because of breakage due to a lack of moisture.**

We have dry hair by nature and every chemical we put on our hair dries our hair out more. There are several things that must be remembered when wearing any chemically processed hair:

- Constantly replace lost moisture by washing the hair frequently

- Use a moisturizing product daily

- Do not brush hair. The chemical process weakens hair and brushing promotes breakage.

Breakage is caused by dryness and abuse. Dryness can be minimized by moisture replacement. Maintaining a relaxer in the weeks ahead is very important because the hair tends to be very dry and easily damageable if handled improperly. Proper care means washing once every three days to one week, with daily moisturizing and deep conditioning with the conditioner described in Chapter 6.

Below I explain how I care for my relaxed hair and the various stages it goes through in the weeks following my relaxer. You may find your hair responds quite similarly.

Weeks 1-2 The first two weeks after a relaxer, my hair has very little body and often hangs limp. In addition to following the advice outlined in this book, these next three points are crucial during this period.

- Wash it a minimum of every three days

- Moisturize daily

- Condition weekly for approximately 20 minutes with **Ultra Black Hair Conditioner**

Weeks 2-4 Continue to wash, condition, and moisturize as scheduled. During this time period, the hair will regain a lot of its natural body and look filler when styled.

Weeks 4-8 In addition to washing, moisturizing, and conditioning, up until the beginning of the 6th week you may elect to just curl your hair immediately without straightening with the curling iron. During this time period I feel it is necessary to straighten my hair with the curling iron from six weeks on until my next retouch to prevent snarls and excessive tugging on my hair, which can cause breakage. I also have about three quarters of an inch of new growth, which without straightening, can be quite difficult to comb.

Weeks 8-10 and beyond Between the 8th and 10th week if I can get this far I am definitely ready for a retouch but hair can still survive if you comb carefully and wash and condition once every three days to one week. Apply a moisturizer daily. I am not advising you to stretch relaxed hair to 14 weeks but it can be done without extreme breakage if you are careful. Frequent washing and conditioning are necessary in order to keep it soft. This is not a requirement and how often you have a retouch will vary with how manageable you feel your hair is.

Combing your hair too hard or too close to the scalp is not advised and can snap the hair between the new growth and processed hair where it is the weakest. Washing every third day will not allow it to dry out as much, and if the hair is straightened with the curling iron you can avoid excessive stress and tugging when you comb it. I strongly recommend using the curling iron during this period to straighten the hair for ease of combing and to minimize breakage.

Relaxer Precautions

The fact that Black hair is very fragile because of its dry condition is repeatedly mentioned throughout this book for a reason. Relaxing dry hair is very damaging and extreme care must be taken to preserve it once it has been relaxed. One recommendation that cannot be stressed enough is to be very careful when having relaxers. Avoid doing your own relaxers and retouches if at all possible. It is easier for someone else to see your entire head, and easier for him or her to wash it out if it starts to burn your scalp.

Do not wash your hair before getting a relaxer or a retouch because the pores of the skin remain open for 24 hours. When the chemical is applied, burning and irritation can occur on the scalp. The scalp can actually be so burned in some cases that scabs appear! If the product begins to burn your scalp within a short time after application, be sure to speak up and request that the chemical be removed.

Exercising just before a retouch or relaxer can be equally as bad as washing your hair because the pores are opened to sweat. I made this mistake once and ended up paying for a retouch that did not have time to work. The chemical began to burn badly and had to be removed immediately. It was not the hairdresser's fault so I felt obligated to pay the bill, but three weeks later I had to return to have the new growth retouched completely. I chose to wait three weeks for fear of not wanting to reapply the chemical too soon because of unnecessary increased drying.

Never relax hair that is brittle, dyed, or bleached. If you question how much breakage is too much before you can relax your hair, consider the next statement. If numerous broken hairs are on the back of your shirt and shoulders when you comb your hair, then your breakage is extreme and having a relaxer at this time could be a serious mistake! Wash your hair with a good shampoo specified for dry, damaged hair, then condition with the conditioner described in Chapter 6, and moisturize your hair twice a day for about three months to minimize your breakage before you attempt to relax it. Should you proceed before your breakage is minimal, you can expect to lose a lot more hair than is necessary!

Do not attempt to relax curl styles! The structure of your hair has already been changed once and relaxer products must change the structure again. Over-processing occurs and results in breakage. Remember that these two products were not designed to work together and putting one over the other can severely damage your hair to the point where it will break and fall off at the weakest part of the hair, usually where the new growth and previously processed hair meet!

Common Problems With Self-Relaxers

Two common problems (excluding poor rinsing) that are often experienced when you attempt to do relaxers at home are over-processing and inadequate comb out.

Each relaxer products instructions contain a chart for timing different hair textures depending on whether your hair is fine, medium or course/resistant. I always thought my hair was hard to relax. When I initially attempted self-relaxing, I would always keep the relaxer on for the maximum time period. When I finished, my hair was very dry and extremely brittle and I never knew why. When I began having it done professionally, I was surprised to learn I have medium textured hair. According to the timing guide, the product was only supposed to be left on the medium texture time period, not the maximum.

In June of 1989, when I could not afford to go to the hairdresser for a retouch, against my better judgment I decided to do one on my own. I chose a product off the shelf at the local department store and applied it as I had watched my hairdresser do. After rinsing my hair I found I had forgotten to comb the product through long enough on the left side of my head. Breakage was more apparent as each day went on and my hair became extremely dry. I thought my entire plan to write this book was sabotaged because I feared losing my hair.

Although my attempt at my own relaxer was disastrous, it was also a blessing in disguise. I remembered that protein was the only thing that can actually strengthen the hair by becoming part of it, so I immediately rushed out to buy a protein treatment. After the very first application I realized the importance of protein for dry, damaged hair. Instantly my breakage was halted! This was also a revelation because I realized that protein was the final necessary element we need for growing longer, beautiful Black hair!

Chapter Summary

1. Avoid doing your own relaxers unless you feel it is absolutely necessary.

2. Use protein products to strengthen relaxed hair or any hair that has been chemically processed.

3. Moisturize relaxed or permanent-curled hair daily.

Summary

Over the past 10 years people have sent me comments to incorporate in my book. This is not a picture book so I will never fill it full of pictures. Sisters who want to grow their hair want information. Consult a stylebook if you want pictures. I added more source references so people would not dismiss this hair care strategy as an opinion of the author. I have revised ideas and expanded on my original research findings. Most of the original information remains unchanged because it was true back then and is still true today!

When I first started writing about Black hair in 1989, there were no good references to cite. Now 11 years later, there are lots of good books that address our hair, whichever way we choose to wear it.

I try to keep abreast of what the hair care industry and other professionals are saying about our hair. Two books I recommend you read are *Andre Talks Hair* by Andre Walker and *Don't Go Shopping for Hair Care Products Without Me* by Paula Begoun.

Andre Talks Hair by Andre Walker – I enjoyed Andre's book as it gives a great explanation of the 4 hair types. I never knew how to explain what type of hair I have until Andre identified me as a Type 4. There were some things in his book that I disagreed with, especially the use of brushes and "feeding the hair," but it is still a very good book.

Don't' Go Shopping for Hair Care Products Without Me by Paula Begoun – I referred to this book several times. Paula's research was extensive. There were some issues I disagree with her on, and I am sure she will also disagree with me, too. Paula did not review my products, but based on what she has said about others there are ingredients in my products that she speaks against using. However, my products work well for me so I stick with them. My products and methods have successfully been tested for over 10 years!

I do hope you've enjoyed reading my book as much as I have enjoyed writing it. You can master successful hair growth whichever way you choose to wear your hair. Using this system with any hair type will help you keep your hair and add length.

The $6 billion hair care market manufactures products from basically the same ingredients. The use of adjectives like: texturizing, revitalizing, volumizing, clarifying, replenishing, moisturizing, and hydrating are expected to appeal to your emotions. Stop expecting to find a genie in a bottle. Good results don't have to be expensive. The magic of Black hair growth doesn't come from a bottle. The mystic is removed when you learn how to care for your hair. Growth comes when you put forth effort.

Let your approach to hair growth be common sense.